Anyone who has cancer or who has relatives or friends with cancer must read this book. It is insightful, compassionate and funny - and packed with useful information and practical ways to handle everything that comes up from the side effects of treatment to the staff in hospital. I can't recommend it highly enough.

JUDY HALL, *'Crystal Bible' 1, 2 & 3*

Margaret Cahill offers the reader the opportunity to walk with her hand-in-hand on her journey returning to health and well-being, where she offers the simple yet profound advice to 'become your own expert'. From blog to book, here is proof that we are all 'editors' of our own stories.

ANITA MOORJANI, *New York Times bestselling author, 'Dying to be Me'*

This is a book of Hope, Strength of Will and Spirit. A book that defied fear and refused to accept defeat. When faced with months of chemotherapy the author turned for support to her family and to the friends who knew her well. Through the medium of a regular blog she shared her good and bad days, the highs and lows, the dark and light moments as she slowly turned the tide against the internal foe. Every woman should read this saga of courage, humour, and love of life. If it has happened to you, let it give you hope; if you have never had to face this enemy, give thanks and bless those women of courage who, like Margaret, fought and won and those who are still fighting.

DOLORES ASHCROFT-NOWICKI, *SOL*

Cancer happens in the dark. Beneath our awareness, deep within, it builds its citadel, and we only discern its presence as it reaches its zenith. Margaret perfectly articulates what it means to make a struggle in the dark against this unseen, but keenly felt enemy. With wise insights and heart-wrenching humour she leads us along a struggle where life was always her first choice.

SWAMI AMBIKANANDA, *Founder, Traditional Yoga Association*

As a cancer sufferer myself for more than a quarter of a century (two terminal diagnoses and counting) I recognise the real thing when I read it. Margaret Cahill has the courage to tell it how it is (and how it may be if one confronts the illness proactively, and without damaging preconceptions). Her book will horrify some and comfort others. It will guide those with the wit to listen, and reassure those embarking on their own dark night of the soul that they are not alone.

Through all the many vicisstudes of her treatment Margaret's true nature shines through. The cancer did not change her - it simply reinforced her already existing essential self. May her experiences, and the grace, elegance and humour with which she confronted them, serve as lessons to us all.

MARIO READING, *bestselling author of the 'Antichrist Trilogy', and acknowledged expert on the prophecies of Nostradamus.*

The feedback and suggestions from the many blog contributors on nutrition and alternative therapies make this book an invaluable source of information for cancer patients and their caretakers. Since the author is a Mind-Body-Spirit publisher, her authors and blog followers (many of whom are experts in their fields) offered myriads of suggestions ranging from diet and crystal therapies to positive thinking and visualisation techniques. Not only is this book an inspiring survival manual for cancer patients, but its humor and objectivity make it a choice read for anyone who enjoys real-life drama and pathos. Highly recommended.

BOB MAKRANSKY, *author of 'What is Magic?', 'Magical Living', 'Thought Forms' and 'The Great Wheel'*

Not many people journey to hell and live to tell the story. Those who do rarely give us insights on how to avoid hell or deal with it. This is the strength of this book. A must-read for anyone dealing with cancer or anyone who has loved ones dealing with it. It will save lives.

JOE POLANSKY, *Diamond Fire Magazine*

The joy that runs through this book may well give hope and indicate, possibly, a path that others may take, if facing similar challenges. Margaret shows how meaningful illness can be, and the psychic depths that could never otherwise be explored with such intensity. Her story shows illness to be a gift, though it takes some courage to think of it that way.

WANDA SELLAR, *author of 'Directory of Essential Oils', 'Introduction to Medical Astrology'*

An amusing and poignant book that will touch your heart whilst also making you laugh out loud. Margaret writes from the soul, allowing you to fully experience a journey that most would keep to themselves. She approaches it with dignity, strength and humour. Brilliant!

JENI POWELL, *Director, Crystal Healing Academy*

Under Cover of Darkness

How I Blogged My Way Through
Mantle Cell Lymphoma

Under Cover
of
Darkness

How I Blogged My Way Through
Mantle Cell Lymphoma

Margaret Cahill

BOOKS

Winchester, UK
Washington, USA

First published by O-Books, 2015
O-Books is an imprint of John Hunt Publishing Ltd., Laurel House, Station Approach,
Alresford, Hants, SO24 9JH, UK
office1@jhpbooks.net
www.johnhuntpublishing.com

For distributor details and how to order please visit the 'Ordering' section on our website.

Text copyright: Margaret Cahill 2014

ISBN: 978 1 78279 930 6
Library of Congress Control Number: 2014959594

A CIP catalogue record for this book is available from the British Library.

Printed and bound by CPI Group (UK) Ltd, Croydon, CR0 4YY, UK

We operate a distinctive and ethical publishing philosophy in all
areas of our business, from our global network of authors to
production and worldwide distribution.

Contents

Acknowledgements

I have been dreading writing this. How can I possibly thank everyone who has helped and supported me through this cancer journey without missing someone out? However, I do want to try as there are some public acknowledgements – in no particular order – that I think are very necessary:

Swami Ambikananda: Thank you for your constant and sometimes harsh love, which has always been there for me. You have the magical knack of always being at the end of the phone when I really need you. Thank you for always speaking the truth to me, however much I might not want to hear it.

Manisha: For solid and profound dietary advice back when all this started, and ever since. You are the reason for mystified doctors and why my mouth never, ever got sore from the chemo.

Cathy: The heroes (and heroines!) who work behind the scenes often don't get the recognition they deserve when in fact they are the people who keep it all together when a crisis hits. Thank you from the bottom of my heart for dealing with all the words when you really wanted to be safely back in figures-land, and for single-handedly keeping The Wessex Astrologer going in my absence. Thank you also for my lovely pink wineglass. Richard, you probably don't think you played any part in this at all, but actually you did, and it was massive. Trust me.

Lyn and John: Thank you for being the quiet strength that kept Stephen and me going through the darkest times. For driving us to the hospital at a moment's notice, for getting Stephen back on the road, for lovely sunny coffee mornings in your garden, and for providing much needed hilarity along the way. You are both precious beyond belief.

Judy Hall: For providing endless love, crystals and healing, and for never failing to accompany me on journeys into the darkest recesses of my mind. Thank you for taking us around Egypt in photo form and for presenting us to the ever-powerful Egyptian gods and goddesses in order to facilitate my healing; for encouraging me to undertake the 'Weighing of the Heart' ritual despite my fear, then rejoicing with me at its lovely outcome; for being constantly strong, and resolutely convinced I would survive this.

Jeni Powell and Guisseppe: For giving me so many beautiful healing sessions and the opportunity to benefit from the new crystal matrices you were testing out. It was an honour to be your guinea pig.

Komilla Sutton: I will always treasure your phone call from Delhi airport. A test of true friendship, as you were talking sense that I didn't want to hear. Throughout the years you have always been a calm and strong support, and you were quite right – we can keep in touch just as easily wherever you are living. Your mum is amazing and very special too. Big hugs to you both.

Dr. Emma King: For giving me the worst possible news at the beginning of all this in the gentlest and kindest possible way, then escalating me up the theatre and scan lists as fast as humanly possible; for delivering the best possible news in December 2014 when we discovered that my fears of it all coming back were foundless.

Dr. Joe Chacko: I think any consultant would feel they got the short straw having me as a patient. You deserve a medal for keeping me in a treatment regime I had never planned on being part of, and that I fought all the way. Thank you for listening to me and Stephen when you really didn't have the time, and for allowing me to embrace both East and West in my treatment, all with the most amazing smile. Most of all, thank you for giving me back my life.

Lisa Hammond: The stem cell transplant was always the 'biggie', the elephant in the room that would eventually break loose. Thank you for sneaking it up on us then guiding us through the whole thing and making it as bearable as possible. Your infectious laugh and the brightness you bring into any room made a huge difference.

The staff on Wards 10 and 11 at Bournemouth Hospital: My respect and gratitude for the astonishing level of your compassion knows no bounds, including of course the wonderful Dot. After I stopped being scared of you I realised you had a heart of gold and would leave no label unread in your quest to help me get the food I wanted. Thank you also for letting me take over your fridge with strange coloured liquids.

Kris Brandt-Riske and Jack Cipolla from the American Federation of Astrologers: The pink hats! What more can I say? We were touched to the core at your thoughtfulness and incredible timing – and for the continued support. You two are the best.

Dolores Ashcroft-Nowicki: I am honoured to have been included in rituals by the Servants of the Light. Your constant faith in my ability to survive this has been an integral and vital part of my healing.

Jennifer Staveley-Hall: Thank you for making it so easy to talk. And we can certainly talk! Your wisdom is so far beyond your years, or possibly this lifetime; Steve, thank you for always being loving and so supportive every time I called for yet another marathon session with Jennifer.

Zsuzanna Griga: For supplying the gorgeous bath oils that helped me retain my sanity in my 23 day incarceration. The rose-filled bath on transplant day was symbolic beyond belief.

Sue Joiner: For running and inviting me to the totally nutty Village Writers' Group in Brockenhurst; for staying in touch and posting such beautiful, heartfelt comments on my blog; for including me in your prayers.

Jonathan Taylor: For creating such a stunning cover and for being a totally splendid graphic artist and all round lovely guy. Thanks also to Shanta for your idea for the white lines on the cover.

Terrie Birch and Tore Lomsdalen: For escorting the photograph of me and Stephen to the sacred sites along the Nile in order to facilitate my healing, and for taking such astounding photos of us as we 'visited' them with you; for allowing me to use the pictures on the blog and the cover of this book.

Garry Johnson: For taking such gorgeous photographs at the wedding of my lovely niece Natalia and her hubby Mike Leonard, and for allowing me to use the main picture on the cover. You achieved that rare thing - a good picture of me!

Barnaby Roberts: For being the catalyst that started this whole thing off. The full story is given on p. 46 as it would take too much space here, but suffice to say, you are one very special person.

Darrelyn Gunzburg: For your totally brilliant idea of writing the blog to keep everyone updated. You have literally changed my life by opening my eyes to the joys of writing.

Bernadette Brady: Our lovely long (chilly and cold!) walk along the beach was amazing and a balm to my soul. Thank you for your unshakeable faith that I would get through this.

My amazing family, including: My older brother David, currently residing in France, for endless Skype chats about the meaning of life and all that stuff; my oldest son Ben for supplying me with the infamous 'dongle' which allowed me to stay in touch with the world and for sorting out my iPod again and again as I'm not good at this stuff; Matthew for sending me crazy videos and pictures to keep me laughing even when I was too ill to have visitors; my beloved Stephen, for never shying, for one moment, from the horrors we faced and for holding my hand all the way through the tears to the sunshine at the end.

For Stephen
My light at the end of the tunnel

Introduction

Judy Hall

Light becoming

I feel both very honoured and very grateful to have been asked by Margaret to write an introduction to this amazing book. Honoured because it is a remarkable testament to the courage not only of an extraordinary woman but also of her partner Stephen and all those who supported her journey, and grateful to have been part of the process and to still have this wonderful friend and publisher here with me as we continue to move through her expansion. This book is yet another step along a soul-expansion journey I believe she set in motion before arriving on this planet of ours. Margaret has always been there for me, as a publisher and as a good friend, so to have the opportunity to be with her as she journeyed through her darkness was a privilege – and a pleasure. A strange thing to say when some-one was facing such a life threatening illness but the way she turned it into a healing challenge was a joy to watch. I never doubted that she would survive, but I knew she had to go right to the edge and beyond in order to be reborn.

"Where did that come from?" were the words with which I greeted Margaret's announcement that the consultant she'd hurriedly been sent to see had diagnosed lymphoma. Not at all the caring compassionate response I'd have wished to make. But it does reflect the absolute shock of the diagnosis and how it came out of the blue – and, unknowingly at the time, some underlying questions as to why that I intuitively sensed. I was convinced that this was not karma but rather an opportunity for soul growth that she had programmed into her journey. Yes, I knew she'd been having trouble with tonsils since she came back from what one of my friends referred to as 'the sinkhole of the world' because of its toxicity on so many levels. But cancer? Margaret? One of the, seemingly, most healthy and active people I knew? A woman who had only recently found a relationship that would support and nourish her after a series of shambolic episodes. I had envisioned her finally living the life she craved. Now both she and the relationship would be tested to the limits.

I'd been there at the start of that relationship. Might even be said to have given it a nudge. I was in the office discussing the launch party for my book *Good Vibrations* when Stephen rang. We both knew him as the manager of Watkins bookshop and editor of *The Watkins Review* (now *Watkins Mind, Body, Spirit* magazine) but had never actually met him, so I said "ask him to the launch party." And then, a little later – because a voice was whispering in my ear "this is the one she's been waiting for" – "ask him for his birth details." It's a good job it wasn't a Skype call as Margaret put the details into her computer and then compared it to her chart. The huge grins, gasps and "look, look's" that were going on at our end as we compared the charts and looked at the relationship possibilities between them bore no relation to the calm and measured tones in which she was discussing the delivery of books with Stephen. But when she finally put down the phone, we hugged and did a jig around the office and by the time they met at the launch, the outcome was a foregone conclusion. A relationship made in heaven, twinflames if ever I saw them. Twinflames offer each other mutual support and room to grow, a bit like what most people think of as a soulmate but they are here to help us learn lessons rather than be with us as we go through a growth process (see my book *The Soulmate Myth* for a definition and the rest of the story.) I am convinced that without the unflinching support of Stephen, Margaret never would have made it through. He too is an extraordinary person and I honour him.

Margaret was born under the zodiac sign of Cancer and, when I teach about that particular sign, I always point out how caring and nurturing the sign is and how intensely private. That crab's shell conceals a great deal. So when we discussed the idea of her blogging I knew that this was a challenge for her, and yet it gave her the opportunity not only to pour out her heart with true humility and enormous humour and compassion, but to let her readers walk alongside her and watch her soul growing. I'd always known she had a book to write, I just hadn't thought it would occur this way and, clearly, neither did she. But there is more to how I teach about the sign of Cancer. Years ago on a television wild life there was this cute little hermit crab that had got too big for his (her? how do you sex a crab?) shell. It sidled up to a few prospective new homes, sideways of course because that's how crabs approach things. It looked terrified at the prospect of moving, eyes darting everywhere. Eventually it found one it liked. It approached a few times, even walked around it and put its head inside, but backed off again and again. You could see the battle going on "should I, shouldn't I, dare I?" Eyes out on stalks it looked longingly at this new home – if that's not anthropomorphosising a crab too much – but I swear it had desperate desire in those eyes. Then, rather than going right up to the new des res, it did a rather remarkable thing. It heaved itself out of its shell, wriggling and pulling and puffing and panting. It really had stayed in there far too long and was all but stuck. With one extra effort, suddenly it was free although naked and highly vulnerable. It scuttled across to its new home. But as it did so, a remarkable thing happened. It grew to twice its size. As it settled into its new home you could almost hear the sigh of relief and feel the pure joy that was emanating at having successfully made the transfer. There are rather a lot of predators out there only too happy to snack on a shell-less crab.

Why am I telling you this? Because when I first saw Margaret after the diagnosis she looked just like that little hermit crab. Wide eyed and terrified. Totally vulnerable. Not surprising given the suddenness and seriousness of the diagnosis. All I could do was hug her. But even then she was up for doing some healing work and digging deep inside herself. A process that continued throughout the next few months when she was shell-less, only in her case the predators were her own rogue cells and the chemo that was to destroy them but in the process decimated her immune system. No wonder she needed to take all the home comforts into hospital, so Cancerian. They usually lug bags of possessions along with them although Margaret had been remarkably free of that tendency prior to that. Working with the Egyptian healer-god Imhotep throughout her illness was another privilege that took me places I'd never been before and brought me some amazing experiences and connections. So it was with great joy that I saw her after the stem cell transplant as her hair began to grow again and her eyes were shining with joy not fear. She'd come through. Her compassion and open-heartedness were so great that, when I temporarily lost virtually all my sight, she and Stephen were the first to do a food run for me – the bags of goodies were most welcome as was their company. And then the remission was declared. A new, much stronger, woman emerged from the ordeal. Comfortable, it would seem, inside her own skin, just like that regrown hermit crab.

One of the healing rituals that we undertook with Imhotep was a death and rebirth. Margaret did eventually decide to include my reply to her post in this book but I'm also including it here as a tribute to one of the most incredible women I have had the privilege to call friend.

Dearest Margaret
It was a privilege to walk through the Duat alongside such a light, lovely and courageous soul. How could you ever doubt that your heart would pass the test? You give so much joy to everyone. I have no doubt at all that you will safely make the same journey now through the physical level of this incredible experience into renewed life. Regenesis – becoming Isis. A true initiate, you represent wisdom, immortality, life, fertility and knowledge for us all. You are an inspiration.
Heal well
Mega hugs to you and Stephen
Judy

Prologue

New Orleans, Louis Armstrong airport, May 2012. We stepped out into the atmospheric equivalent of a hot, wet blanket and made our way over to the winding queue for a cab. By the time we had gone all of the 15 feet needed to get there I was soaked. Short of going into a steam room, I have never got so hot and sweaty so quickly in my entire life. Given that I'd usually go into a steam room wearing just a swim suit, to say that after a flight from London I was overdressed would be no exaggeration. Jeez.

My partner Stephen and I were in New Orleans along with over 1000 other astrologers for the week-long United Astrology Conference, being held in the prestigious Marriott Hotel in the French Quarter. As a publisher, it was a brilliant opportunity for me to network as well as meet up with a whole bunch of my authors; ironically, most of them are from the UK, and we always joke that we have to fly halfway round the world to actually get to see each other. Such are the wonders of electronic communication. It still amazes me that I can work on a book with someone for months and get really close to them – editing someone's much treasured manuscript certainly gets you up close and personal – but maybe not get to meet them in person for years. Or ever!

So – we arrived at the hotel in a jet-lagged fashion, abandoning as many layers of clothing en route as was decent. We were given a great room with views over the Mississippi, and for once I was glad not to have a balcony as the humidity would have defeated me in seconds. Working on the basis that we should stay up until it was a sensible time to go to bed, we changed into as little as possible to go out and explore and find something to eat. Jetlag adds a really special dimension to your senses. Combine that with a couple of glasses of wine and being in one of the craziest and most buzzing cities I have ever seen and I wasn't sure whether I was hallucinating. A jazz band played on the street, just around the corner from our chosen restaurant, where we had taken a table out on the pavement. That was a silly decision, but as you can tell, we hadn't yet acclimatised and we assumed the evening would become cooler. So wrong. From our ringside seats on the pavement we watched all kinds of humanity pass us by. New Orleans is hot and especially steamy, in every sense of the word. Prostitutes were doing deals literally right in front of us, there were stag night parties wandering by with the guys carrying full sized blow up dolls around their necks, transvestites strutting their glorious stuff up and down the street... it went on.

New Orleans never cools down. Atmospherically it is always hot and very humid with the result that you dive from your very cold air-conditioned hotel into the wringing wet outdoors then into your chosen, almost certainly air-conditioned destination as fast as possible. I was busy taking the mickey out of the – um – 'unfit' guests from the hotel who were taking a cab two blocks, until I tried walking it myself. Horrible, and absolutely my idea of hell. It was cabs after that wherever possible. I was also finding it very hard to adjust to the time change and was beginning to dread every night as I would lay wide-eyed and very awake for most of it, despite my usual arsenal of sleep aids.

We were being hosted at the conference by the very lovely Kris and Jack, on their stand for the American Federation of Astrologers, who distribute our books in the USA. During the day I was meeting current and potential authors, and most evenings Jack and Kris made sure that Stephen and I were entertained with brilliant company, fantastic food and copious amounts of wine. Even the wine didn't help me sleep and as the days passed I was becoming more and more depleted and just wanted to get home. Much to my annoyance I started to get a really sore throat. We travel well-stocked with natural remedies for this kind of thing. And I mean well-stocked! We had tea tree oil, grapefruit extract, Echinacea tablets, lavender oil, Quiet Life plus all the usual painkillers. One notable afternoon we took some time off to explore; as we came out of the hotel we realised it was raining, and no, we hadn't thought to pack an umbrella. We wanted to catch one of the trams running from the stop in the middle of the road so thought we'd risk it – after all it was only a shower. Oh no it wasn't. The heavens opened in a totally non-negotiable fashion and we found ourselves running across a road that was rapidly turning into a torrent. By the time we got to the tram stop we were absolutely dripping. Literally. We made it onto the air-conditioned tram and stood in a state of freezing drippiness until our stop, where we alighted to – sunshine. See? How nuts is that? We walked around in the sunshine until we were dry, at which point we became too hot and had to retreat to the freezing interior of any air-conditioned shop that would have us. Are you starting to get a feel for the climate? This is no doubt beginning to paint a really gloomy picture of our trip. Yes, there were amazing nights out to gorgeous restaurants, the wonderful jazz band in the traditional jazz club, the boat trip through the swamps where Stephen held a baby alligator, the ride in a horse-drawn carriage around New Orleans, the gorgeous dress I bought at a totally ridiculous sale price… there were many things that were good. However, by our last full day, when we decided to take a steamboat trip up the Mississippi, my tonsils were so swollen and sore it felt as if I was swallowing razor blades. I had used all our painkillers and we had to buy more to get me through the day and then – home.

My first stop once we got home, was of course, the doctor. We had been back a few days and by the time I got to her I had bronchitis as well as tonsillitis. She didn't prescribe antibiotics (she knew how much I hated them) and seemed confident that with sleep and rest I would recover. A few weeks later and I was back at the surgery. My tonsils were still fighting my uvula for space in my throat and I was exhausted. I was also desperate to get back to work as although our bookkeeper Cathy had done a sterling job of keeping the office going in my absence there was an awful lot to catch up on. So I came away from my second visit clutching a prescription for antibiotics. They didn't work, and neither did the next lot I was given several weeks later. By now I was aware through the wonders of Facebook that other people had also been ill after their trip to New Orleans – ranging from colds and flu to asthma attacks. What was going on? Obviously the climate had got to other people too.

Several more visits to the doctor followed and I was eventually sent for blood tests. It was about October by now and despite a luxury cruise in the Mediterranean I was clearly far from well. I called for the results of the blood tests and was told by Reception that my blood counts were normal and that although one of them was slightly raised (the lymphocytes!) the doctor had signed them off and didn't need to see me. I felt kind of abandoned. I was obviously ill but with nothing to prove it. I tried some tincture for tonsillitis from my favourite medical herbalist, colloidal silver (which for some reason my body really hated), crystals, meditation, any and all kinds of healing, hands on and remote. I posted on Facebook and found out that everyone else who was ill from New Orleans had recovered. I also discovered around then that my right tonsil had taken on a more alien appearance than the left one, which was just plain swollen and red, so I went back to the doctor. He is one of those thoughtful types who leans back in his chair and looks at you. He did a fair amount of leaning back thoughtfully, then said, "It does look jolly odd, doesn't it? I think we'll get those chaps over at ENT to have a look at you," and made an online appointment for me for 11th December. In the time between my visit to him and the hospital appointment I went to the surgery twice more as I felt so ill. A blood test for the Epstein Barr virus also came back negative.

December arrived, and with it our Christmas party. After years of paying through the nose for hotel functions where the food is appalling and the music is stuck in the 80s, we decided to hold our own black tie affair at home, with my son Matt, who is a musician, providing the entertainment. This particular year we were also blessed to have a friend's daughter sing for us. Her voice is truly one of an angel and she had the whole room in tears with her rendition of *Pie Jesu*. The idea of having a black tie party was to get the guys out of their jeans and t-shirts and to give the ladies a chance to dress up – and it worked really well. By this stage I was going home from work early as I didn't have the energy to keep going all day, and I was really worried that I wouldn't make it through the party. With the help of a rest and a belt of distant healing however, I survived and we had a beautiful evening.

That was Friday 7th December, and I had actually started to get a bit of a Christmas spirit. We did some Christmas shopping at the weekend and I almost managed to forget about my forthcoming appointment.

By the time it came, I was, actually, almost flippant. I was so used to feeling ill and being fobbed off that I didn't have high expectations for a useful outcome of this appointment either – to the point where I was quite happy to go on my own, as Stephen was so busy with deadlines for the *Watkins Mind, Body, Spirit* magazine for which he is the Managing Editor. By several strokes of intuition I asked him to come with me, and I am so pleased I did.

The consultant, Dr Emma King, was absolutely lovely and ruthlessly efficient. Within 5 minutes she had heard my story, pushed a probe up my nose so it would light up my throat and felt all my lymph glands. And told us she was 90% sure we were dealing with lymphoma. Really weird things happen in your brain when you are given bad news: denial, you think you've misheard, you don't believe what you have just been told. The cogs turned slowly in my mind, and I remember feeling somewhat stupid as I asked, "Lymphoma is cancer, isn't it?" "Yes," she replied, so gently.

Stephen and I huddled together in stunned silence as she started to make phone calls. Where she got voicemail she tried another number until she found a real person, calling in favours to get me an appointment for a full body MRI scan the next day, and adding me onto an already oversubscribed theatre list for a biopsy/tonsillectomy on the following Monday. At that point we didn't know which it would be. We left the hospital in shock.

I feel as if I cried for days, and through it all, Stephen was there to hold me as our world and our future disintegrated before our eyes. Because that is what a cancer diagnosis does. You can be the most positive person in the world – and I like to think I am some way up that scale – but knowing you have a disease that will kill you without some kind of dramatic intervention makes all your plans for the future look very wobbly indeed. Telling my sons was horrendous and I now have an understanding of what my mum went through when she discovered she had breast cancer. Giving the news to loved ones was doubly bad as everyone else was getting into the party mood ready for Christmas and I felt as though I was raining on their parade. My niece phoned, full of excitement, to discuss our family get-together planned for Boxing Day and I had to cut across her to explain what was going on. She was incredible and immediately offered to help pass the news on as by this stage we were more than sick of the 'c' word and all it implied. Dealing with your own shock and grief as well as the reactions of other people is very tiring and upsetting, and there seemed to be no relief from the horror of it all.

The day after the appointment with Dr King I was back at the hospital for a full body MRI scan, and I was whisked through the milling crowds in Reception straight into the scanning suite like some kind of medical royalty. It was almost embarrassing and I started to picture millions of cancer cells invading my body in a surreal race against time. Surely it couldn't be that urgent.

Stephen and I spent the following Monday as guests of Poole Hospital Outpatients department. I had been asked to starve from the evening before and to be at the hospital for 8.00 the following morning. It was like one of those bizarre dreams where everyone else knows what they are doing except you. Droves of people were being checked in then herded off in groups to other areas, except for us. This happened several times and I eventually asked the nurse when I would be called. At first she couldn't even find my name, then it turned out I was on a different list. All the other folk were in for minor procedures but I was on the list for the senior consultant as they didn't know what they were going to find. And there were two people before me, one of whom would be having a four hour op. Wonderful. The nurse wondered why we had been called in so early, and after checking, said we were free to go into Poole town centre as I definitely wouldn't be called for a few hours. That was also bizarre. The shops were full of Christmas cheer but we couldn't have been less interested – at least it used up some time though and took my mind off my hunger pangs, which were by now becoming pretty insistent. We got back to the hospital just as some of my fellow patients were coming back from their procedures and being released into the care of their relatives. I was SO hungry.

I was finally called at 3.30, by which time we were on first name terms with the nurses, the helpers, the cleaners... you name it.

The surgeon decided just to do a biopsy as he didn't want to disturb too much tissue, but thankfully he took away enough that my uvula could now function properly. In recent weeks my tonsil had been firmly pressed against it which was very uncomfortable and was also causing my voice to change. It also meant my recovery time would be that much quicker than if I had a tonsillectomy. I wanted to be well enough to go ahead with our Christmas as planned, as far as possible.

In the Beginning

Talk about being thrown headlong into 2013... I have to say, never in a million years did I think that I would be preparing for our Christmas party on 7th December then taking a call less than a month later to be admitted to a cancer ward. I imagine everyone has the same feeling when they get the dreaded diagnosis of cancer, so this blog is going to be my journal as I find my way through a very different landscape to the one I expected in 2013. Stephen and I have been touched and even overwhelmed by the support that has poured in from more people than we realised we knew, and it is already impossible to keep everyone updated with the latest news. My hope is that we can use this blog to keep everyone updated – please do feel free to post in reply. It will be lovely to stay in touch....

We got through the Christmas period with the love and support of our fabulous families and friends, knowing that in the New Year treatment would start in earnest. In fact, we had the love and support of far more people than we realised. Stephen and I both know a lot of people through our work, and word spread fast. We found we were spending long evenings on the phone repeating the same story to many different people, as well as sending texts and emails until we were absolutely sick of the whole thing. After 2nd January the action really kicked off, and it became impossible to keep everyone updated. A very dear friend expressed upset at not being included in the loop, which in turn upset me, so at the suggestion of one of my authors I decided to start a blog. It was very strange being on the writing end of the process; as an editor with over 15 years publishing experience in my own company, I am much more comfortable working with somebody else's precious words than baring my soul through my own. It turned out to be a life saver. Not only did it serve its purpose and provide a place for friends to go for updates, it allowed me to work through a lot of the stuff that was, and still is, going through my head. I started writing in a diary but I soon realised

I needed a much bigger forum for my thoughts; the blog was a living entity as readers could post their own comments, all of which were kindly, very supportive and usually thought-provoking. I could read and comment on them in my own time, and I was absolutely loving writing each blog.

I was stunned by the response and by the feeling I had when I was writing. It was amazing to 'liberate' my thoughts – that is exactly how it felt – and I seemed to be hitting the spot with the people who were reading:

From Bernadette Brady:

I am glued to your blog and thank you for letting us into your journey. Much love.

From Darrelyn Gunzburg:

So glad you are doing this blog. The title is fabulous. Your journey will be extraordinary. We will walk with you now every step of the way. Have trust and faith in the process and be of good courage.
Much love. xxx

From Neil D. Paris:

Margaret, just stopping by to let you know I am with you in spirit through your journey, and I'll be checking in here to see how you're doing. You'll be getting massive beams of Light from this end! Few things for you – I used to always stay away from conventional medicine too but have come to learn that some things we do need extra help with on the physical plane and the help has really been beneficial. Also, I have always believed too that illness was a spiritual imbalance but then through my own adventures now I am open to the possibility of it just being another challenge, another quest our soul signed up for and therefore there is no blame and no imbalance, just another life experience to experience, absorb and transcend. Only the strong ones get the biggest challenges, right? Your Virgo Moon and Pluto have a new focus, a new project. A spiritual upgrade, perhaps. Margaret 2.0! ....I love you, and I believe in you. To the journey!
Neil xx

Very soon they started to ask whether the blogs would be turned into a book at some point, which was incredibly humbling. I really was just pouring out my thoughts every week or so; a book? That was a whole new ballgame that required a lot more thought.

That thought, at the time of writing this chapter, had been tumbling around for a further nine months, so it seemed an appropriate time to start giving it some structure. I had reached the end of the course of treatment and there was an insistent clamour in my head for all this to be discharged in some way. The irony of that word has not gone un-noticed! Organising it all has been challenging. Each blog seemed to pour fully-formed from my mind after about a week of gestation, and as it acted as a diary for the previous week I thought there wouldn't be a lot more to add. Also, the blogs usually developed a theme while I was writing them so in a way I was unwilling to interrupt that flow by breaking them up or editing them to fit neatly into a book.

In a sense the blogs, when joined up, tell the whole story. But they also don't. A cancer journey is far more than 1500–2000 words poured out once a week. There were whole back stories going on that never got a mention, as well as massive rollercoasters of emotion, and I wanted to give voice to them as well. I eventually decided to leave the blogs pretty much intact and to write around them; alongside the cancer treatment they formed the structure of my life for nearly a year, and became my way of getting through some very difficult times. Once I started writing them, I found that I looked for the quirky and unusual moments in my experiences so that I could relay them to 'my readers', thereby giving a very mundane and boring event a bit of interest. I could also chronicle my battles with mainstream medicine and bureaucracy, knowing I would find a receptive audience. After all, I had to go through them – why not share the misery?! I can't begin to tell you how much that helped me to cope.

So here we go. Here's how we were plunged into a brave new world:

... Mantle Cell Lymphoma is a very aggressive and rare cancer, and to stand any chance of survival I need to have equally aggressive chemotherapy which will see me pretty much out of action for the next 3-5 months. I usually stay

well away from conventional medicine but this is non-negotiable. I will take the best from all forms of treatment that are available, conventional and alternative, physical, emotional, psychological and spiritual. I have some very dear and gifted friends who are advising me on the supplements to support my system as it is ravaged by the chemo, and I have a truly wonderful consultant who is taking advice from the leading expert on treating MCL. I am in good hands. I'm going for my PET scan on Monday – that's the one that will make me glow in the dark :-) – then on Tuesday I go in to have the Hickman line put in. Early Wednesday I start the chemo.

Stephen and I are just taking each day at a time. There is no other way for us at the moment as the bigger picture is too difficult to deal with. Our dear friend Judy Hall commented on the unusual name of this cancer – a mantle usually covers something, and she wondered what could be revealed from this experience. I do believe there is a spiritual imbalance which is at the root of physical illness, which is why I have called this blog Under Cover of Darkness. *In the hours before dawn everything does indeed appear very dark. But just as the Sun rises to bring light into our lives each day, so do I look with hope and optimism towards a revelation that will help all of this make sense to us.*

The response was overwhelming – love and good wishes poured in from all over the world, both as comments on the blog and via emails and texts which gave us a massive boost. I always used to play my cards fairly close to my chest, but writing the blog was a huge lesson: if you have the courage to open up, people will take you to their hearts. Within days we had become part of healing circles and groups, and the feeling that we had a deep well of support was to nourish us through the long cycles of chemotherapy that lay ahead. The title of the blog also attracted interest.

Our dear friends Lyn and John has this to say:

As a matter of interest Lyn and I have a couple of paraffin lamps (showing our age), just in case we cannot afford the electricity! In their centre they have a mantle. This acts as the element and provides the bright light that alleviates the darkness.

Well, I never knew that!

My initial two-day stay in hospital for tests was horrendous. I felt as though I had been pitched into somebody else's nightmare, only I didn't seem to be waking up. The first day was taken up with being admitted, having blood tests and trying to absorb the fact that I had cancer as well as various visits from doctors, including the lovely Dr. Joseph Chacko. We were given information sheets and told that a treatment plan would be discussed the following day. Stephen left for the evening and I faced a long, cold night in an isolation room.

Most of the rooms on Ward 11 are in isolation as cancer patients are very vulnerable to infection. I was bitterly cold and didn't sleep at all. I discovered that the TV screen had internet access, and in the wee small hours did the worst thing possible: I looked up Mantle Cell Lymphoma. I read that less than 3% of tonsular cancers are lymphoma, and of those only 5% are MCL, which is considered incurable. Of those 5%, 95% are men over 60. Where the hell did I fit into that profile? Worst of all, median survival rates are 5-7years. Judy later told me (something I had never considered, in my misery), that the reason survival rates are given as 5-7 years is because that is the only data currently available due to new treatments being developed all the time. I have since discovered that with the advent of stem-cell transplants the survival rate is much better.

However, at 7.00 on that dismal morning I was busy sobbing my heart out in sheer terror at the enormity of it all, when a lovely nurse popped her head round the door to see whether I wanted breakfast. Her shift was finishing but she sat with me while I cried, which was a long time. Somehow, the feeling that she had seen it all before really helped lessen the shock and horror in my heart – at least, temporarily; she told me that there would be tough days, but there would also be good times. And mostly to remember that there are no medals for bravery on a cancer ward. It is somewhere to let it all hang out whenever you need to. Naomi rapidly became one of my favourite nurses.

I certainly did that. I managed to force down some Readibrek (the only un-sugared cereal available), but everything fell apart when Stephen arrived. I couldn't tell him all the awful things I'd discovered and yet I had no doubt that he had looked it up too.

I was busy sobbing again when the door opened and Dr Chacko walked in. Seeing how upset I was he came round to hold the hand on the other side of the bed from Stephen, and sat down. He held it all the way to the end of the visit. I was so heartened and touched by that gesture. From that point onwards and probably in contravention of all medical hierarchy he became just 'Joe'.

Almost immediately two more doctors came in, followed by the Senior Staff Nurse. It is bad enough being upset in private, but a continuously increasing audience is beyond tolerance. When the door opened again to admit yet another doctor, my sick humour finally broke through: "Please, just start without me. I'll be right there."

I discovered that this whole multi-doctor meeting around the bed thing is called 'Ward Rounds' and it happens twice a week. I fairly soon wised up to the politics of it, especially with other consultants, but with Joe at the helm it was always very productive. He wanted me to have a bone marrow biopsy that morning to check whether the cancer had spread, as well as an echocardiogram to make sure my heart was healthy enough to withstand the enormous toxicity of the drugs I would be having. I would be following the Nordic Regime which involves six cycles of chemotherapy three weeks apart, followed by a stem cell transplant. That was the next six months sorted then. I was also to have a PET scan, which would show the extent to which the cancer had spread to other organs, if indeed it had. My chemo would start the day after the PET scan. I was discharged later that day to await the appointment.

Hospitals are strange and life-changing places, and I don't know the exact statistics, but I would guess it's not very often in a good way. Being turned out into the bright sunshine, blinking through my still-flowing tears, I had no idea what to do with myself and my thoughts. Being a very 'do-it-now' kind of person, it is very hard to sit around waiting for a phone call for a scan appointment that will show how close to death you are. Or how far away, of course, but I wasn't feeling especially positive at that point. What I was able to do though was to throw myself into work and start cranking up some kind of support system for the company for the duration of my treatment. All the books we were working on had to be put on hold. Creating a book from a manuscript is a very intensive process, and it isn't fair to the author to string it out for months on end. Ironically we were working on *Judy Hall's Book of Psychic Development* at the time; Judy had been a close friend to Stephen and me for years, but she truly came into her own from this point onwards.

There were office practicalities to be dealt with – everyday activities that I do as second nature – but passwords and PIN numbers had to be written down, Idiot Lists and instructions recorded for the use of anyone who happened to be in and could help fill orders or pack boxes. A business doesn't run itself; it is an organic and ever-changing beast that demands constant attention and regularly throws a strop if ignored for too long. After more than 16 years of running The Wessex Astrologer I was not about to see it fail, cancer or no cancer. I am sure this was a great support for me but at the time it felt like a huge weight on my shoulders.

Enter Cathy the unflappable. As our truly stunning book-keeper she is priceless, but she really does prefer dealing with figures rather than words. She willingly stepped many leagues further than her comfort zone and turned her hand to whatever needed doing at the time. The plan was that a) there was no way I was going to ever be in hospital for as long as Joe had said and b) I would stay in touch via my laptop so I could still read company email and support Cathy where possible. The planning and implementation of survival tactics made the days pass quickly, and in no time I was facing the PET scan, followed by my first cycle of chemotherapy. The whole scan debacle is covered in my second blog.

Crazy Day

Blog #2 14th January, 2013

Crikey. What an odd day. After having to forego breakfast for this procedure, I was expecting to progress through the PET scan unit in a hungry but sedate fashion and then go on to do a huge amount of work at the office before I signed off for chemo.

The universe obviously had other ideas.

I made it to Southampton hospital with a few minutes to spare and proudly reported to the mobile scanning unit ahead of time. The staff explained that the scanner was having some checks done so they were running a bit behind schedule. I had about half an hour reading Gareth Malone's Choir then was called to have the injection which would send a radioactive marker and glucose belting round my system. The nurse inserted the cannula so they could give me the injection more easily – getting so used to all the needles that I didn't even register the 'sharp scratch' they like to warn you about. She explained that once I had the injection the staff would keep their distance – fair enough.

She wasn't kidding. I was shown back to the cold little cubbyhole that was my 'rest area' and waited for a while. A few minutes later the door was flung open and she rushed into the room with a metal box that was beeping in a loud and very alarming fashion. This was beginning to feel a bit like a Denzel Washington film. In less time than it has taken me to write this sentence, she opened the box – bleeping got louder just to hurry her along a bit (I think it also flashed red from inside but I'm not completely sure about that) – took the end off the device, injected the liquid through the cannula, closed the box, removed the cannula whilst simultaneously sticking a plaster over the wound, then ran out calling over her shoulder, "You're all done, I'll be back in an hour."

Wow. I expected to start glowing, or feel at least somehow different. I've never been radioactive before (at least not to my knowledge) so I was very interested to see what would happen. Nothing.

I had about 45 minutes more of Gareth then the nurse sidled back into the room and from the corner explained that the scanner was in fact broken so they couldn't scan me today. I sat there for a moment waiting for it to make some sense to me. So what were they actually going to do with this (by now) very hungry and highly radioactive person? Actually there must have been several of us at this point, all sitting very confused in our little cubby holes wondering what the rest of the day would hold for us.

When my wits returned, I explained that I needed to be scanned today as I am starting chemo tomorrow – so I could go somewhere else if there was another scanner available. She suggested Portsmouth, which is about another 25 miles on from Southampton. I left several minutes later with a map to the hospital and the stern instructions, "Get there as fast as you can. And don't go near any babies or pregnant women as they could be harmed by your radioactivity." Sooooooooooooo. Hospitals have a fair amount of babies and I did have to go past the maternity ward on the way out, so I had to kind of skulk past people pushing buggies and was horrified when I nearly brushed by an expectant lady. I reached the car (which by now seemed like my refuge) and hurtled out of the multi-storey car park. The car park takes you out a different way from where you go in. People who know me well are constantly amused by my ability to get lost anywhere and today was no exception. I have no idea how Southampton is laid out and I was very quickly lost.

Bearing in mind that as I was radioactive I couldn't exactly go into a shop to ask directions (don't have satnav – well I do have an iPhone but the battery was unexpectedly flat), I managed to accost a postman, at a distance, to get directions back to the motorway. Several minutes later I was happily and hungrily belting down the M27 towards Portsmouth hospital. It did occur to me that if I went very fast I might attract the attention of the police and maybe I could even get them to escort me with the blue lights and everything. Can you imagine the conversation?

"And why exactly were you going so fast, madam?"

"Well, officer, I'm highly radioactive and I have to get to the hospital as fast as I can…"

In the end I decided the sedate approach was probably better and would take less time in the long run. And less explaining. I reached the hospital in good time and was rushed through the reception area. I felt really sorry for the people who were also hungrily waiting, as they were being told they would have another two hours before they would be seen – the escapees from Southampton had arrived! It seems that three of us had come straight from there and the lovely folk at Portsmouth slotted us in with only about ten pages of Gareth in terms of waiting time. After that it was plain sailing.

The actual scanning took about 45 minutes. It wasn't too claustrophobic, but I was getting quite fed up with playing statues by the time it finished. I was back in the waiting room by 2.30 and sat down to enjoy my 'breakfast' of slightly warm cheese sandwiches. Made it back to the office by about 4.00, so needless to say we didn't actually leave to come home until about 7.30.

The lovely thing about today was that when you are in this kind of situation, you just have to go with the flow. When you give up any sense of control, life becomes much easier. This is quite a lesson for me as I am a total control freak – and I suspect the coming months will be an in-depth study in the art of giving up the illusion of control. Accepting what comes. I have no choice about the fact that I am now ill, but what I can have some control over is my attitude and my approach to dealing with this illness. Today was fun in a really weird kind of way – I met some lovely people and had quite a few laughs at the absurdity of the situation. Long may it continue.

Thank you to all of you for your beautiful words. I am touched to my deepest core at your kindness, and I will carry it forward with me into hospital tomorrow and thereafter.

Needless to say this went down a storm with my fledgling audience. And I was beginning to find some sort of flow in the writing, and releasing my thoughts on such a horrendous situation into an amusing blog was very liberating.

From Sue Joiner:

Hello Margaret,
I couldn't catch the blog address on my phone. Thankfully Judy has emailed it to me. Hearing loss is such a nuisance but I can tell I am about to see that's all it is.

Looking at your blog from a reader's point of view, this has been quite something, very absorbing, brilliantly upbeat. Although I'm a horribly earnest creature you made me laugh – several times. There can't be many with the ability, the wit, and the will to produce something like this.

From a writer's point of view you'll know how 'lucky' you were to have had this extra 'drama' on the first day!

From a personal point of view – not! But from now on if you find yourself in another OMG patch think of us the readers; one in 3 or is it 4 of us, is going to have to face something like this. And certainly most of us will know (or will have known) someone else going through a similar experience. Some of your readers will be saying in recognition 'Yes, it is (or it was) like that! Your family, friends, colleagues, and those connected to fellow patients (strangers to you perhaps?) will gain insights which they can pick up and revisit when they are properly in a position to absorb them. And not just them; there are the medics (and hospital managers!) who, for all our sakes, also need these insights.

Is that a euphemism for truths? No; an insight is surely a deeper truth. But in this instance the standard truth will be quite enough for anyone – that while indisputably ill, you had to dash irradiated from one hospital to another (how many miles?) because the (one and only?) scanner had broken down. Not too many could make a laughing matter of that.

Now I will take another hopeful look to see whether you have written some more!
Love Sue (J)

From Fei Cochrane:

Hi Margaret,
I am very proud of you. You are such a strong and extremely brave person to handle such a situation alone. Good Job. You're such a wonderful model for all of us. Hang in there and continue to be strong.
You are always included in my prayers.
Love, Fei

People were going back and reading them historically too, which I found pretty incredible.

I had this lovely comment from Deb Houlding:

This post is nearly 3 months old as I read it. I know it shouldn't, (since I'm aware of the seriousness of your condition), and yet it makes me smile. This is life – crazy, chaotic, dramatic, but also comedic, even in tragedy. I haven't read what happens next, but am hooked on your story Margaret – the thought of you panicking out of concern of passing your radioactivity onto others epitomises why the human condition is so glorious :).

To which I replied:

Lol. I think that is what keeps me sane. If I stopped too much to think about what I'm going through I would just give up. There are dark moments, to be sure, as you will no doubt find out as you read on, but there is always room for laughter, isn't there, even if it is just at the absurdity of the human condition in all its technicolour glory :-).
M xxx

Absurd indeed. And it had only just started. We arrived for my first chemo session in the style of a Sherpa train fit for an expedition. Following my freezing night in isolation I was told I could bring my own duvet, in fact my own anything, really. So I did. Several black bags later I was settled and ready to get started. One thing I would come to realize is that hospitals are there to get you better as fast as possible so you can make a speedy exit. They are not there for warmth, comfort, good food, or internet access.

Just a Quickie

Blog #3 16th January, 2013

I love all your comments and I am so pleased you are enjoying my musings. I am having problems getting the wi-fi sorted out here. Apparently I need a dongle. Is it just me or is that word a bit dubious round the edges? It sounds as if it should have a backing track of schoolboy sniggers. Anyhow, I should have said appendage tomorrow and as long as it behaves itself I will be able to upload a new proper-sized blog without too much more delay. We do have touch-screen monitors next to our beds with internet but I'd say that definition is circa 1980. 'Smack screen' or 'thump screen' is probably more descriptive of the manoeuvre required to produce a line of text. But I was willing to put up with the pain and possible risk of RSI just to stay in touch. Finally start chemo tomorrow but more of that little hiccup with the next post. M x

The lovely thing about writing for a truly international audience is the misunderstandings and general hilarity that occur on a fairly regular basis.

Kris Brandt Riske from the AFA chuckled along with me:

LOL! Okay, for the somewhat uncivilized Americans (like me and Jack!) reading your blog, what's a "dongle"? Is that a password? A "backing track of schoolboy sniggers"? Great phrase that I will use in the future... once I know what it means! Much, much good luck and good thoughts for today's first chemo. xoxo

To which I replied:

Yay, back online!!! With my somewhat temperamental dongle. I really thought someone was joking when they mentioned a dongle. I assumed it was the equivalent of a widget or 'thingy' but no, in this context it is a mobile broadband device you plug into your laptop that connects you to the internet wherever you are. However, I think it does also mean 'plastic thingy' because I have two dongles on my Hickman line, to which I am now firmly attached, with all kinds of toxic chemicals pouring into my system. Oh well. That's life. Still think dongle is someone having a laugh at our expense. If anyone on here knows better do enlighten us!

This kind of humorous support was exactly what I needed, as there was indeed a hiccup. Chemo didn't start the next day either, as my sometimes erratic heartbeat decided to kick off. More of that further on as it is quite a special little story which appears in a later blog.

On this first day I was taken down to have a Hickman line fitted. It is inserted under local anesthetic (some people had a general anesthetic but that involved not eating for six hours – no way!) on the right hand side of the chest, and magically plumbed into the vein just under the collarbone. This stretches the skin a lot and for the first few days it is really sore. The other end emerges a few inches further down and just above the right breast, as a white plastic tube that divides into two 'lumens' which are used to give injections but are also great for being on a drip; I would be attached to drips for hours at a time and it would be far too painful to have them administered through a cannula. The lumens themselves have to be flushed with saline solution before and after every use and at least once a week. (Even with all that attention they can easily become infected.) The line is held in place under the skin by a thickened 'collar', around which the tissue eventually grows. This contraption might be useful medically but it was to become the source of much irritation, both physically and emotionally. My next blog revealed how I saw the rest of my 'settling in period'.

Settling In

Blog #4 17th January, 2013

With the trauma of my trip to Southampton and Portsmouth rapidly becoming a distant memory I am now writing from my hospital bed; yes, I made it! I never thought I would actually be anxious to get admitted to a cancer ward, but it is strange how a sense of urgency pervades one's thinking. Knowing that I have an aggressive cancer makes me panic for every moment that it goes untreated, even if that treatment is likely to make me very poorly indeed. Veteran cancer survivors will probably chuckle at my inexperience, but it is very odd to be told that something silent and deadly is growing inside me – which as far as I am concerned didn't even exist before 11th December.

There is something amazing about the human spirit and its capacity for survival; whatever the situation, there is a primal instinct that draws us together in times of danger. We become a clique, a special club. Was it Groucho Marx who said that he didn't want to be a member of any club that would have him as a member? He hadn't been on a cancer ward. I was welcomed with smiles and kindness by everyone, and I feel very safe. Safe because I will be receiving the best medical care possible (apparently Bournemouth General Hospital is renowned internationally for its cancer care – result!) and safe because here I can be funny and scared by turns as the emotions arise.

Scared especially of Dot, who runs the tea trollies and delivery of meals. Yesterday (um…Wednesday I think – completely lost track of time) Dot was pretty grumpy because the night staff hadn't been round to change the water jugs before they went off duty. Which they do – oh – around 6-ish if we are lucky. Apparently it used to be 5.00 until the patients formed a posse, safely armed with plastic spoons, to request just a teeny bit more sleep if that is at possible please if it fits in with the schedule. Well they won that battle but I don't fancy their chances in winning any war against Hospital Routines. It's funny how new situations bring out one's lack of confidence. Anyway, I'm not that great at speaking up for myself and on my first afternoon here Dot asked if I'd like a cup of coffee. "Oh yes, thank you. I'd love a cup of your very special economy, headache inducing, powdered instant coffee please!" No, joking. But I did say I'd like a mug of white coffee, no sugar please. At least the drinks stay warmer in a mug. The cups are specially designed for hospitals so that the drink is cold by the time it reaches the recipient. Can't risk people spilling cups of hot tea over themselves as that would reflect badly on the Health and Safety figures. So Dot wanders back to the trolley repeating 'black coffee no sugar' to herself. Have you spotted the difference yet? This would only end in one of two ways. And she would win both of them. She came back with – yes! – a black coffee. I hate black coffee. Maybe I would have to drink it. (She wins.) Was I brave enough to correct her? Nope, I'm a wimp in these situations. (She wins.) So I politely asked if I could have milk after all, and she shuffled back to the trolley muttering that I had asked for black. At least I got out of that one intact! The coffee was grim though...

The whole philosophy of being in hospital is really quite interesting. I'm not ill in the normally accepted sense of needing bed rest and constant care, but a lot of the people in here really are. We get amazing medical attention but there is no peace, no sense of stillness in a busy day, which is what people need in order to get better.

I am currently in a two-bedded ward in the isolation unit (because that is all that is available just now). The lovely lady I am sharing with is very sick. She had a blood transfusion yesterday, something she has had about every three weeks for the last two years, because in her form of cancer her own immune system is attacking her body and it is destroying her white blood cells. There is no known cure for her condition, but her consultant is leaving no stone unturned in the quest to find something new that will help. After every transfusion she is exhausted. Even I can see that she is desperately tired and yet she is given no peace. Blood pressure check at 6.15, woken again at 7.00 (and lights turned on – we turn them straight off again!) for a cup of tea she doesn't really want. Immense hassle this morning at just after 7 when Dot was cross because nobody has ordered their lunch yet on the in-house system. I did speak up that time as I was really cross. "Fifteen patients and nobody has ordered their lunch yet!" she says. This is about two minutes after the lights have gone on. "That's because we were asleep, Dot," I bravely venture. "Fifteen patients and it has to be in by 9.00!" "That's because we were asleep, Dot," working on the scratched record basis

*that something might sink in if I say it often enough. It doesn't. Breakfast
follows at 7.15, more drinks at 8.00 and then the bedding is changed and
tablets handed out. A tiny oasis of peace then the doctors come in to do their
ward rounds. Then it is time for more blood pressure checks. My lovely and
very poorly room mate has just got back to sleep having told everyone she is
having a lazy day (like she needs to make an excuse?) when a student nurse
appears to check her weight. There must have been about 20 minutes of
blissful silence before the next interruption: the counsellor wanting to check
that she is OK after being a bit upset the other day. NO SHE ISN'T. SHE
NEEDS TO SLEEP.*

*As a relatively healthy person (I am still convinced I am too well to be
sick) I am already exhausted by the relentless interruptions and busy-ness
that pervades the hospital. I am typing this as the cleaner is moving my bed
around. If I leave this laptop for too long without paying it any attention it
goes into sulk mode, so as she said I could stay on the bed I am. Quite fun
really, up high with the guard rails out so she can clean underneath. Oh no.
She is going to my roommate now, who has just got back to sleep!*
More soon
Mxx

I felt curiously like an observer out on some kind of special assign-
ment. That mood was obviously coming across in the blogs as Reina
James (one of my authors) had this to say:

*You seem to be next to me here, talking! I can really hear your voice and see
the ward and dear Dot. We're thinking of you, in your wellness, dancing gor-
geously on some lovely shiny floor. And also trying to get a moment's peace...*
Love and hugs from us to you and Stephen,
xxxx R&M

Support was also coming in from other cancer sufferers. Mario Reading, a member of the afore-mentioned Village Writers' group run by
Sue Joiner and a very successful writer himself, was diagnosed with
terminal cancer about 20 years ago. He is a lovely, vibrant guy with a
rich sense of humour who is very much alive today, despite the odds.
He had this to say:

My goodness, when I keep (kept) my hospital diaries they were really diaries
– we had no blogs then. And now I'm just in the habit of keeping hand-writ-
ten diaries. I think blogging from the hospital is a brilliant idea, and your
blogs are excellent. And you are 100% right, Margaret, to remind them all
that you are a person and not a number! The few times I have ever really
gotten angry in hospital are when they forget that – I remember lecturing
a whole roomful of French interns once about just this. Anyway, I'm really
glad my note was a help. I'm off myself to the Royal Marsden soon (they're
going to experiment on me with a new trial drug which I fear may turn me
green or something similar). Remember this: everyone will tell you you are
sick. But if you don't feel sick, then you AREN'T sick!! Then they can do
what they want and it can't touch you. And now I'm going to say some-
thing that is going to sound a little daft. But try to love your cancer. It is
an integral part of you, and is not something you must fight. You will only
exhaust yourself. Love it. Accept it. And then, with a little luck, it might
clear the hell off out!!!
xx Mario

I was delighted and really touched that he had commented:

Hi Mario,
Thank you for your kind comments – they mean a lot coming from you.
It is odd that I don't feel the need to fight the cancer. My dear Swami-
ji reminded me that the way to freedom is through acceptance – if you
fight something there will always be the threat of a battle that may well
be lost, and as you say it is exhausting. I feel I need all my strength to
move through this in ways which are only revealed to me on a mo-
ment by moment basis. I am sure you know that one. I would love to
chat to you when I get out. Should be coming home tomorrow so when
I have slept the sleep of the sleepy I'll get your details from Stephen.
Big hugs
Margaret

Judy also commented:

What Mario said about loving your cancer is an interesting approach –
and one that's served him well while living with 'terminal' cancer for 20
years. You know how amazing and full of life he is (his blog at http://blog.

marioreading.com/blog/ is fascinating and so full of insights). Maybe seeing the rogue cells as naughty schoolboys who've got out of control and need to become more disciplined and stop wreaking havoc would be the way to go? The drugs are rounding them up and putting them in detention until you can restore order and show all parts of your body that they are loved and cared for? Opening the earth star chakra beneath your feet and your base chakra would help with the meditation, grounding you in your body so that the healing power can flow in and assist the drugs. Just a thought... worth a try.

Despite the painful Hickman lines and the hospital routine, I was still convinced I was totally well and shouldn't be there. At this point I hadn't actually had any chemo so I also felt like a fraud. That was about to change though as the next day my treatment started late, but in earnest. The fact that it started late meant that it would finish late – I wasn't aware of the implications of this when I suggested we push ahead rather than lose another day. I grew much wiser very quickly and for future treatments did all I could to get them started earlier.

5. Getting Started

It has been a long and frustrating week in some ways, seemingly dogged by delays (medical) and technical difficulties. But we are finally at Friday and I had my first chemotherapy treatment yesterday. It lasted from 12 noon until 1 a.m. this morning and was non-stop toxic chemicals flowing into my system through the IV. Curiously, one of the most distressing things was the background vibration of the pumps pushing the drugs in. It seemed to permeate into my very bones, and possibly made me feel sicker than the drugs. Well that was what I thought until this morning :-) Give it up for anti-nausea drugs!

More of that in a moment. Rewind to the previous evening. Hospital time exists in its own continuum, and whoever dreamed up the schedule needs a good slap. I like to think I am more of a morning person than a night owl, but I find drinks at 7.00, breakfast at 7.15, lunch at 12.15 and tea/dinner at 5.15 all a bit much. It feels very much as if we are rushed through the system to suit working hours of the (very lovely) ancillary staff at the cost of a more sympathetic and natural timescale. 8.00 arrives and it's all over bar the shouting as this is when the last drinks trolley of the day comes round. Now – the lovely night nurse gave me the most fabulous up-to-the-minute news the other night, considering this might become my second home for a while. She asked me what I wanted to drink. Fatal. It's good to get out of this Rice Krispies, turkey pie, fruit cocktail kind of existence once in a while (is it ever good to get INTO it?!) so I couldn't help myself. I just couldn't stop it coming out – ingrained habit, sorry! "I'll have a nice large glass of cool Chardonnay please."

To give her credit she absolutely cracked up and so did the other lovely lady who had just ordered her tea – and clearly thought she had missed her opportunity to get something a bit more exciting. Apparently at Christmas the doctors organised a drinks trolley on a couple of days, and in their infinite wisdom – and they are all-knowing, right? – they decided to instigate a Sunday night drinks trolley. Result! Shame I might be discharged by then, but I'll be sure to place my order early when I'm next in.

It is now the day after chemo so I have time to reflect on my first serious brush with Big Pharma. I usually avoid doctors and drugs as far as possible but in this situation I very much want to live using whatever resources are available, as opposed to die by my principles. I felt my heart sink as I read the enormous list of chemicals that would be given: for every drug that kills the cancer there has to be another which will alleviate its toxicity. It was the strangest feeling, watching bag after bag being pumped in; I was grateful to be in the hands of experts but upset at the invasion of my body. I tried to meditate during the IV process and be accepting of the moment but the drugs made me feel very woozy and sick. Going up to the place where I usually meditate was really uncomfortable and ungrounded so I had to stop.

I was talking to one of the nurses about this conflict and she told me of another patient who sees the drugs as good soldiers who have come in to kill the bad guys. It was suggested to me that I could add the condition 'and do as little harm as possible', which makes a lot of sense. I am hoping I can get to a place of acceptance – and less hostility – towards all this, as the important thing in the end is that it works. It is a very big lesson for me and I am gently tweaking at the edges of it to find out more. I do have many dark moments, and it is healthy and a recognised stage of grieving to allow the anger out. There is a growing feeling of why this, why now and of course, why me? I will never be the same after this. For any cancer patient there is always the shadowy threat of regression from which you can never be free, and that has fundamentally changed my thinking.

Today (Friday) I am pumped full of more drugs in preparation for discharge, and to be honest I will need a supermarket trolley to take them all home. Which will be tomorrow!!! My blood tests are all back and fine so I'm outta here. Until next week when I come back for a blood count check.

For those of you who followed my madcap dash across Hampshire for the PET scan – we just got the results and it is clear. Relief is too small a word for it. There are apparently a few weird teeny weeny lumps on my head but they can look at those when my hair all falls out, which will be in about 10 days. Much too much hair around at the moment to see anything. See – always a silver lining!

And guess when my next treatment starts? A Thursday. Which means... I will be still be in on the Sunday for the drinkies round!

Fortunately my sense of humour was still prevailing. Judy helped when she posted this:

Can't wait to see you in a fluffy pink hat to match your duvet cover and towels holding that glass of Chardonnay. Good timing for the next visit. Heal well xxxJ

I replied:

Hey yes! Good suggestion! The isolation wards are really cold so I will need a hat... so it obviously has to be pink. They all loved the duvet cover and slippers, and Fenella Flamingo (pink of course) attracted attention. One of the nurses asked why I stopped there and didn't carry on to a shag pile rug. Hmmmmm... :-).
Mxxxxxx

Nevertheless, this was my first treatment and my first real insight into life in hospital. I was desperate to get home and out of the clutches of the medics and their endless interruptions as fast as I could, as well as having some decent food for as long as I could stomach it. I knew from my research that supplements would go a long way towards helping my body cope with the toxic onslaught, but I had decided to follow Swamiji's advice, and wait for my body to tell me what it needed. It certainly did that!

I first met Swamiji in 1986. I was looking for a yoga teacher and saw her card pinned up in the reception area of the acupuncturist I was visiting at the time. I called to make an appointment and loved her on sight. A strong and feisty woman with endless depths of love in her eyes; the kind you can fall into, knowing you are safe. At the time she was just called Ambika, a bramacharian monk hailing from South Africa, but now living with her family in the UK.

We bonded immediately and have remained friends ever since. I studied yoga with her for years and she gave me acupuncture while I was in labour and was present when both my sons were born; after my parents died she said she could never replace my mum but that she would always be there for me. And she has been. We shared something we called the 'what next?' feeling. Got married but something is missing – what next? Children. Had the children, what next? Changed job, what next? Doing more yoga, more meditation, started shiatsu, still not enough. What next?

I had access to the amazing array of gurus and swamis who came to stay with her on their visits from India, and who gave generously of their time to her friends and students. The years passed by and Ambika finally took sannyas to become a swami, a Hindu initiation of the highest level only undertaken after many years of deep intro-spection and preparation. We talked several months after her initia-tion and I asked about the 'what next?' feeling.

"It has gone,"she replied. "I have reached the right place."

Swamiji has seen me through the hardest times of my life, but occasionally with some pretty tough love. There were some horren-dously dark times both after my parents died and after my divorce, and I remember her saying that sometimes God does seem to give us more than we can cope with, but we aren't in a position to negotiate. On one particular day I was sobbing my heart out to her down the phone; she gave me a few moments and said, so gently, "You know sweetie, the only thing you can do with this is to open your heart and say, 'Yes. Yes, this hurts like hell, and I don't want it, but Yes.'" That is so hard to do, but I have used it a lot, especially recently. Believe it or not, it really does help.

My body certainly had some messages for me, and I was glad I had listened to Swamiji's advice. I was determined, as far as possible, to get through this experience in better shape than people usually do. I felt I needed to retain some sense of distance and not get swallowed up in the typical cancer patient profile. Easier said than done as it was all a bit of a shock to my system.

6. Life at Home

Blog #6 20th January, 2013

First this from the Sufi poet Kabir:

> *The way of love is not*
> *A subtle argument.*
> *The door there is devastation.*
> *Birds make great sky-circles of their freedom.*
> *How do they learn it?*
> *They fall, and falling,*
> *They're given wings.*

With thanks to Brandon Bays, who quotes it in her lovely book The Journey.

My dearest Swamiji, in a beautiful email I took into hospital with me, told me that I had been pushed off the cliff rather than being allowed to fall gently – which probably comes from pigheadedly continuing on my own sweet way and not listening to the signs I was being given that Things Had To Change. The flying analogy has been cropping up in my life for a while now. Some years ago I had the fancy of writing a book – I had the title but no actual content (pretty typical me, then). The title? Flying Without Wings.

Within The Wessex Astrologer list I wanted to start another imprint for non-astrological books. The name ended up as Flying Horse Books. The idea of soaring with the eagles, reaching for the stars and falling to the Moon and so on has appealed ever since I was first aware of it. I remember my brother telling me as a child (obviously quoting from somewhere or other!), "...and some day Thomas, a man shall land on the Moon", a long time before the supposed Moon landing. No doubt he will tell me where it came from when he reads this!

I now have the chance to fly. Mine and Stephen's lives have changed completely and we have the chance to start anew. Old patterns created a situation in my body where cells turned cancerous, so, as I read in someone's blog the other day, that is a room I cannot revisit. Things Do Indeed Have

To Change. It's really odd when you come back home from hospital. My only experience of any note has been to do with babies. You get the carry-tot seat holding your precious cargo back home, dump it in the middle of the floor because you are too scared to put it on the table – might fall off ?!! – then after a few minutes the sheer weight of responsibility falls with a massive 'thunk!' on your shoulders. It was a bit like that on Saturday, only it was the responsibility of getting me well that fell on my shoulders, and making sure that Stephen survived the process too.

I think it is easy for the caregivers to be left out of this whole process. It has been very difficult to have all the attention directed at me so far, not only because I still don't really believe I'm ill and I hate being in the limelight, but also because I am so concerned about how Stephen is coping with it. He has been working to a magazine deadline whilst supporting me through all the initial hospital appointments, organising hospital visits, bringing me nutritious food to make up for the utter gunk I have been given, holding me when I have needed to cry – and dealing with the extreme and raw grief of knowing I have cancer. I think I have probably said quite a lot so far about feeling blessed and touched by the amount of support we are being given. What is so lovely is that Stephen has very obviously been included in those prayers too. That is so important and once again I thank you all. It is a path we are exploring together; the days I feel well I want to be able to offer any support that he needs and that I would quite naturally have given before – and for us to have fun together. He is not to be my nurse maid. Try telling that to a Virgo!

So we now enter a new room. What are we putting in there? Well, a lot of that hand-cleaning gel that is being advertised, for a start. It is possible, nay, likely, that my white cell count will go down very low in the next few days and I will be very open to infection. According to the MacMillan nurse people are far more likely to be infected by their own germs than those of others – barring shoppers sneezing all over you of course – which includes touching your hair, face, nose, feet, the telephone, computer keyboard. All the things around your home that you use frequently. You can imagine with Stephen's Virgo Sun and my Virgo Moon, we are having a field day!

And we have two cats. I did clear touching the cats and drinking the odd glass of wine with the nurse and I'm delighted to report that both were OK – especially the cats. I'm joking of course. Especially the wine was OK *as she is obviously a woman after my own heart. It becomes a whole new way of living in your own home. It wouldn't be good for me to use the hand towels that the rest of the family use, so I have kitchen towels by the sink. This is nuts. I accidentally scrape my hair out of my eyes, wash my hands, wipe them by mistake on the towel, wash them again, use a kitchen towel. Cat walks by, want to stroke cat as it is good therapy, wash hands, remember to use kitchen towel, wipe hair out of eyes because bending down to cat has made it all fall in my face, wash hands AAAARGH!!! I'm becoming Howard Hughes! I collapse onto the sofa, accidentally move the cat blanket, get up, wash hands... no, I'm being silly now, but you can see we have to get used to this new idea of living in our own home in a way that protects me.*

Protection also of course includes looking at food and supplements. My aim is to try and keep my blood cell count up so I stay fit and am in the best possible condition for Cycle 2. The chemotherapy destroys good cells as well as bad, and as the cells in the mouth replicate fastest these are the ones that get hit first. Thrush (which has already started) and ulcers are a great discomfort so I am taking Aloe Vera juice and vitamin A drops to help. I am using linseed tea to lubricate the whole digestive tract which dries up from the mouth all the way down to the exit point, with very unpleasant consequences. Pomegranate juice is an excellent source of anti-oxidant (and absolutely gorgeous with a bit of chilled water), which along with vitamin D and Echinacea will help to rebuild my immune system. Then there is the vast amount of juicing we are doing. You can see why I won't have time to work.... Fortunately Stephen is joining in with this nutritional programme as otherwise he wouldn't have the strength to keep up with me :-)

We have always been careful about the type of food we buy. I read a while ago that ordinary non-organic veg contains more organophosphates than the legal limit even after it has been thoroughly washed, so quite apart from the fact that it has been grown in exhausted soil which has to be supplemented with fertilizers, we figured that organic has to be best. We have a bit more flexibility in the budget now the wine bill has dropped somewhat, so we are diverting that into the food fund. I don't get along with a vegetarian diet (apparently the Dalai Lama doesn't either so I'm in good company) so we will be continuing to eat some meat. Grass fed animals and fish that are caught from the sea as opposed to farmed will at least have escaped GM grain and antibiotic supplements in their diets. Once you get into all this in any depth it is almost too horrible to contemplate how our food has been messed around with.

Diagnosis of Mantle Cell Lymphoma is apparently increasing at the rate of 4% a year and thus it is likely to become the focus of future research. It is estimated it will become the cancer of the younger generation who are currently filling their faces with poor quality food, and it is directly related to toxicity. I can at least try to make sure that for me and the people I love, there is good, nutritious food available to feed our souls and nourish our bodies. A bit sad about the chocolate though. I'm not a chocoholic but the odd bit is nice. Tried some tonight and the texture was horrible. This is starting to get serious!

Good night!

Margaret xx

The exceedingly grim hospital food had made me focus even more on what I could do for my body in between my incarcerations, and Swamiji's advice was excellent. By the time I left hospital my mouth felt horrible so I started taking one drop of Vitamin A a day, along with two teaspoons of Omega oil. Vitamin D3 drops were also suggested to help rebuild my immune system. Within a couple of days my mouth had improved dramatically, and I stayed ulcer and thrush-free for the duration of my treatment, even through the stem cell transplant. Echinacea seems to be a hot potato with cancer – it is highly recommended by some sources but discouraged by others. We were juicing like crazy, but especially carrots, beetroot, cabbage and celery, with a bit of whatever else was around. Stephen would juice at home then bring me in a fresh batch in hospital. There was a fridge we could use, and my multi-coloured pots generated a lot of interest. Especially from Dot, whose fridge it was. My interest in pomegranate juice attracted quite a few comments from people, ranging from the practical – like just how do you actually juice them, to the symbolism of the fruit itself. All of which was incredibly enlightening.

As Michele Finey, one of The Wessex Astrologer authors commented on the blog:

It is a powerful antioxidant and boosts the immune system. Research suggests it is great at fighting cancer and also heart disease and it has a whole range of other amazing health benefits. It also made me think about Persephone's journey to the Underworld. I have been recently learning how to de-seed fresh pomegranates, which is not an easy task, as you might imagine. This makes sense, with the symbolism I mean, for it is very difficult to separate the seeds from the pulp... Separation and letting go, being such an intrinsic part of the journey to the Underworld. In light of what you were saying yesterday, about control issues etc., when you get home I recommend you explore the therapeutic benefits of pomegranates, both the ritual of de-seeding, and the physical benefits of pomegranate juice! I found that putting the seeds into a tea towel and squeezing the juice out is better than using the electric juicer, releasing much more juice. Fresh is also better than pre-bottled.

I enjoyed telling her about our own experiences with pomegranate juice:

Many thanks for this. We tried straight pomegranate juice when we were in Istanbul a few months ago. We were seated right next to a mobile unit that pressed the juice while you waited. There was at least a pint of it and it was completely fresh and unsweetened. Having tasted the stuff in the shops I was expecting a different experience but not quite as extreme as this! I took a brilliant video on my phone of us both drinking it, which I am going to try to upload just for the laughs. Sucking lemons doesn't even come close! Do you drink it straight?!! I would never add sugar but I wonder if there is another juice that would take the tartness away a bit. We are doing loads of organic juicing at home. Stephen has been bringing me supplies of juiced carrots, celery, spinach, curly kale and beetroot. Classic cancer care stuff which has all the nurses interested. And Dot :-)

Michele suggested adding apple, carrot and beetroot to make it less sour. This blog was proving to be a good support on all levels, and I absolutely treasured the responses it brought. It was enabling me to learn more about nutrition and also to pass my findings on:

Hiya, just heard another interesting thing. A nutritionist and cancer survivor who is helping me with my diet also recommended pomegranate juice, which apparently goes well with whey protein isolate – something I need to take to help build me up for the next cycle. I take it as a very positive sign when ideas from the different areas but with the same eventual focus fit together as they will work more synergistically. Let's hope the taste reflects that!

Michele replied:

Isn't synergy and synchronicity an utterly amazing thing?! It always astounds me when it happens, and I don't know about you, but it seems to be happening more and more frequently of late. Hope you are managing to get your head (and body) around the after effects of treatment.

We had a huge amount of fun extracting the juice using several different methods, all of which created the most humungous mess.

The internal separation process and letting go that Michele and many others mentioned is of course an ongoing and much more complicated procedure. Our good friend Jennifer sent me a copy of *Descent to the Goddess: A Way of Initiation for Women* by Sylvia Brinton Perera, to aid my progress. I turned to it just now to check the details for the credit, and on a whim, did that 'open the book at any page to see what the message is' thing. This is what I found:

We are forced to offer what we hold dear…The sacrifice may change the balance of energy somewhere in the overall psychic system where we did not even want a change.

I certainly didn't want a change. Stephen and I had only just found each other after a long time in the wilderness for both of us, so it was very hard to see what this illness would teach me/us. We had previously done a lot of work on past life regression with Judy Hall – in fact quite a lot of our story is covered in her books *The Soulmate Myth* and *The Book of Why* – and our feeling was that we had finally reached a resting point after a long time of battling with, and learning from life (or lives). We were what Judy calls 'twin flames': without the karma and baggage. Soulmates often have a less than comfortable relationship (whatever form that relationship might take), as there is something between them that must be worked through. There is usually an edge, something that jars, but equally a quality that encourages growth in either or both parties.

This was not the case for us. Stephen and I didn't feel the pressure to grow; we felt we had come home, almost from the first moment we met. A calm port in a storm. A place to get our breath back and relax, just for a moment. Well, it did turn out to be just for a moment, but our deep and very strong connection supported us through the trials that were to follow. As hospital appointments and chemotherapy took over our lives, I thanked the universe on a daily basis that I had someone by my side who was so totally and honestly there for me. No histrionics, no "You have no idea what all this is like for me" tantrums, just absolute, unflinching support. That is a twin flame.

Talking of support, several people had asked if they could add me to their healing/prayer group and if so, to give them a time to 'tune in'. That was weird. It is lovely when people send emails and messages of support, but to officially tell them when to think of me? That was a bit too much exposure for my Cancer Sun. I was still having a hard time of making my illness so public, and this seemed like a bridge too far. However, Judy very sweetly asked me what the problem was in doing so, as I regularly think of other people. Was it that I didn't feel worthy? Ooooh. That one rang true, and, deciding that it was another part of my healing, in the next blog I opened up the armour another chink and gave the good people a time to tune in. It felt very strange, but Tamas, who was giving me very powerful distant healing, told Judy that I had to ask him for healing so that he could reach me. That was a bit easier to deal with. I was becoming a little bit braver about baring my innermost thoughts on the blog – and it was nice to know they were being a) read and b) mulled over.

The ever-lovely Sue had this to say, which really touched me:

Hello Margaret
No doubt there is more to catch up on, beyond this one – I'll go backwards and read that, next, but although it is probably poor taste to say so (Oh when did I ever let that stop me!) this was gripping stuff. I feel absolutely that I have been let in to your innermost self, a self that is original, wise – again probably

inappropriate to say so, because that's not the issue here – talented... and a self that is flying me too, on the back of your... Truth. Honesty – correct, worthy, unilluminated and pedestrian, doesn't have the Universal element. Shared Truths are what we get from memorable poems, and what you are giving us here. If this were transmitted on my car radio – Woman's hour? – at the first opportunity, I would park, turn off the engine, and listen. But now I should be in bed and with any luck you will be reading this after a good night's sleep
Love to you both
Sue xxxx

By way of reply I posted:

Thank you so much for your kind comments Sue – I am deeply flattered. I am really just speaking from the heart. I find that issues arise during the day and I can use the blog to explore them. Writing is so cathartic and I have been longing to write for a long time. Didn't quite expect to be writing about this sort of thing though – just shows that you have to be careful what you wish for!
Warm wishes,
Margaret x x

Practical and very welcome support came in the form of the practice nurses from our local surgery. Chemo depletes the white cell count (en route to destroying it completely just before the stem cell transplant, but we haven't got that far yet), so in an effort to keep us alive during treatment we are given injections of G-CSF (a growth promoting hormone which stimulates the bone marrow to produce white blood cells) on days five to twelve after each cycle. By this stage I was pretty immune to the needles, but had to alternate arms and sides of tummy as they were getting pretty sore. There was the option, oft repeated but never, ever taken up, that I could self-inject.

Absolutely no way.

And in fact just about all the medical staff I consequently surveyed said the same thing, which was interesting and made me feel a lot less inadequate. The nurses who came to see me at home to administer the injections were truly lovely. And to be honest, it was nice, especially in the early stages, to have someone pop in every day to make sure I was OK as very often I wasn't. I still didn't feel 'ill' in the conventional sense and was convinced they were treating the wrong person.

This meant that I was constantly puzzled as to why I might be feeling less than great, and the nurses were great sounding boards who served to remind me that I was on a very harsh treatment regime, and that I should be gentle with myself. I'm not very good at that. If you have a broken leg it is really obvious that you can't go leaping about the place. With chemo, however, you have good days and bad days. And sometimes they can change halfway through, just to catch you out. And I regularly was.

We also had fabulous friends around us who were determined to support us wherever and however they could. Two of these were Lyn and John. Our respective relationships had blossomed at around the same time and we had become very close. What became obvious is that I would be spending an awful lot of time at the hospital in between treatments, for blood tests and consultant appointments, and for those I also appreciated having support – to have someone with me to take it all in, in case I missed a bit of vital information, or forgot to ask an important question. Stephen was working to his magazine's deadline so Lyn came with me for my first post-chemo appointment; I am so pleased she did.

Margaret and Lyn's Big Day Out

Blog #7 24th January, 2013

There is more to life than increasing its speed
Mahatma Gandhi

Yesterday turned into quite a tiring day – possibly the most so far – so I sloped off to bed at a ridiculously early 9.00, abandoning all thoughts of trying to write a coherent blog. And let's face it, the howling rain and wind outside were all the inducement I needed to snuggle up under the duvet with a hot water bottle. Yes readers, a good old fashioned hot water bottle. Right up until all this stuff hit the proverbial fan I have been an advocate of electric blankets, but we are trying to clean up our act here and get rid of some of the more toxic things around our home. And if you are trying to rid your body of toxins it clearly isn't a good idea to be sleeping on a network of highly conductive wiring.

Likewise microwaved and processed food is out. Microwaves lost all their brownie points with me when I discovered two things recently: firstly that in a recent school project, plants watered using only microwaved water shrivelled and died. The plants that were watered with proper tap water did in fact thrive so I don't think you can put the deaths down to the ineptitude of the kids. Sorry. The second is that although veggies might look lovely and crunchy and green (or orange etc.) they actually lose 95% of their nutritional content when microwaved so become, in fact, nutritionally worthless.

Relating this in a circuitous route back to me being ill, it does make me wonder how many of our illnesses are caused because we are not nourished or sustained at a deep level by either our lifestyles or our food. Which brings me SO nicely back to Bournemouth Hospital, and this time to their coffee. I had to go back yesterday to get my blood count checked and my lovely friend Lyn came along to keep me company. Actually she drove me, so it was more a case of being taken, which in the end I did appreciate as it turned into quite an escapade. Firstly, I do have to say that the lady at the WRVS (Women's Royal Voluntary Service) tea bar excelled herself. Lyn's standards for her regulation half-strength latte are legendary, and when we called in for a

40

mid-visit pick-me-up, I did have visions of her being disappointed. As latte wasn't available Lyn graciously downgraded to a cappuccino, which apart from being served in one of those cardboard cups that sticks to your lips, was apparently absolutely fine.

I was under the misguided impression that I would be popping in for a blood test, nipping round to see the MacMillan nurse for some reason I hadn't yet fathomed, then going back home, all in about an hour or so. Oh nooooooooooooooooo. I yet again had this feeling of not quite being part of the club, and someone should really sort this out. The first thing you need to know about cancer club is that you must have Paperwork. Without Paperwork, nothing can happen. Fortunately my name appeared on the guest list for the club, held at the main desk by a very jolly man, who pronounced that yes, I really did exist because I was on the list. That worried me a bit. How many of their patients didn't exist? Or how many really did, but didn't appear on the list? Probably best not to go there in the circumstances. Ward 10 has a special club lounge where guests wait until called for their treatment. Out of date and particularly tatty magazines are considered one of the special attractions here, as is a special ventilation feature. Slightly open window over ragingly hot radiator.

I was soon called for ritual bloodletting. I have said in the past that the staff on the in-patient Ward 11 are absolutely fabulous. Anything really does go and you can be sad or stupid or funny without fearing judgement, which is always going to happen when you are unfamiliar with the etiquette of your surroundings.

Ward 10 has a different kind of code which has a more pedestrian and 'let's get on with it' approach. I sat in the proffered chair and flopped out my lines. (Hickman Lines are inserted above and to the left of the heart and allow direct access into the vein going into the heart. The lines are white plastic, come straight out of the chest and are about 8 inches long. For a lady they usually nestle in her bra. No idea what the men do.) I tell you, for sheer shock factor this knocks the socks off breastfeeding in public and I can't wait for an excuse to do it in M&S.

Fortunately the nurse had seen it all before and she calmly arranged all the test tubes ready to receive my precious blood. We then started on this arse-about-face discussion of when my lines were last flushed. I said, Saturday, when I left here. She asked when the District Nurse was going to do them again. I said on the day of my last injection to boost my cell count, which is 6 days hence. She said that was too far away, they have to be done *Every Seven Days*. I think I know this as an awful lot of people have said it. So I suggested that maybe she do them both today when she takes the blood. Nope. Apparently they only take blood from one line each week so Someone will have to clean the other one at a different time.

WHY?! Why not consolidate? Why not say,"Oh here is a person with slightly grubby lines, could do with a flush, let's get on and do it"? I think I must have looked so stunned at the non-joined-up-thinking going on here that she relented and as a huge favour did them both. Then she asked for my line flushing record. Oh no. I didn't have one of those. "You need to have a record of whoever touches your lines." This was getting perverse and ever so slightly kinky. I'm sure that even porn actors don't get this level of atten- tion. Happily I now have my lines record safely stashed and will make sure I have a signature for whenever anyone so much as looks at them.

The lovely District Nurses have been calling in to give me my cell-boost- ing injections and they mentioned that I could have today's injection done as part of my blood-letting visit. I was beginning to worry about mention- ing this given the debacle of the line-flushing incident, but I had no choice – I had to have the injection.

"No problem", she breezily replied, "have you got the prescription?"

Blank look from moi.

"You were sent home last week with a prescription for the District Nurse so she could administer the injection. Where is it?"

I told her that the District Nurse had it now because – um – it was ad- dressed to her and she took it away to her special place where she presumably puts all the things addressed to her. This meant I had to get the next person I was seeing, the MacMillan nurse who co-ordinates all the treatments (still don't know why I was seeing her!), to fill out a NEW prescription so that I could come back into Ward 10 so that someone could inject me. Jeez. You couldn't make this up. And all this time my lovely friend Lyn was expiring in the club lounge outside.

I was finally dispatched back to said club lounge to await results of blood tests – AHH yes, THAT is why I had to see the MacMillan Nurse. At this point I needed my warm cheese sandwich (yes, another one) and Lyn required fortification with a latte-turned-cappuccino so we repaired to the WRVS tea bar for half an hour.

You'll be relieved, I'm sure, to know that it did all work out OK in the end. My blood cell count is holding its own and Catherine (the MacMillan Nurse) wrote the prescription for my injection, which, curiously, she managed to give me herself, having written and signed her own piece of paper. Not before asking why I was clutching the entire box of injections to my breast. "You should have just taken one out and popped it in your handbag to bring here."

"B-b-b-but I didn't have the right piece of paper," I stammered. Kid you not, I really, really did. Lyn was there and she will vouch for me.

We nearly made it out unscathed after that. We got all the way to the final set of doors, a very good 5 minute walk from the ward, when Lyn remembered that we hadn't stamped the car park pass. Cancer patients get free parking! So we schlepped all the way back through the double doors, up the stairs, through more double doors, along the corridor, sharp left into Ward 10.

"Hello," smiles Mr Jolly, not recognising us. How could he not? We were only there just now. Have we ceased to exist?

"Just stamping ticket and we're outta here!" Phew made it. And next week we do it all again... :-). Thank heavens for Lyn.

Several people have suggested starting a healing circle for me and they requested a suitable time at which to tune in. If you haven't done this before and would like to participate, you just have to sit quietly at the allotted time and send healing thoughts in my direction. Thank you for such a beautiful thought. 21.00 GMT would be good for me and hopefully it is OK with most other time zones too.

Margaret x

Having Lyn around is always like a mobile party, and we had a lot of fun that day, even with all the waiting and messing around with paperwork. What I hadn't realized was that I was gradually becoming initiated into a whole new lifestyle along with its own language. This became obvious when I started talking about the technicalities like Hickman lines. Darrelyn asked me this:

Hi M,
Good to hear the cell count is holding. Yay! Now I know you have valves inserted into you so that it makes it easy to take blood but for those of us

who remain uninitiated, maybe you could explain what lines are and how
they are flushed?
Sending love,
Darrelyn x

I struggled a bit with this so sort of ducked out on the blog and suggested people Google it if they wanted to know more!

I found the Hickman lines an incredible intrusion into the sacred temple of my body. Chemotherapy is a totally de-humanising experience anyway – at least I found it so – because you lose any sense of the natural rhythm of your body. All the usual routines fell by the wayside; my appetite became irregular and unreliable, my taste buds changed, I struggled immensely with the sickness, and diarrhoea was never very far away. The exit point for the lines never really healed properly and the discomfort reduced my mobility more and more. Anything involving my right arm caused the wound to become sore so I just kind of retreated into my body. I felt really ugly with tubes coming out of my skin, and I stank of chemicals. No wonder I had my down days. It is at these times the support from loved ones became even more precious because they just saw it as part of a journey that would see my return to health. That inner pulse of love and strength kept me going through the dark times. Judy was in touch every day frequently recounting what we had been doing together on other planes of existence. My constant desire for pink – a source of great amusement to everyone else – revealed itself to her and she communicated this to me:

I 'dreamt' about you last night. I was sending you healing and I remember
walking up to you and holding out my hands to meet yours. Then we were
in rose quartz. It was most extraordinary. One of my clients had written
to me yesterday about crystalline civilisations and here we were in one of
them. It's the source of the fluffy pink light. I know I've always seen rose
quartz as unconditional love but this was us as part of that. Can't quite
explain, it was like nothing I've done with a crystal before and I've forgotten
most of it because I drifted into the sleepy 'dream'. But I do think you should
have some about your person at all times!

And then…

Yes you definitely need the pink, it's not just a girly reaction. It was really clear that rose quartz was 'you' in a very profound way and it does carry the unconditional love you need to give yourself and to accept from outside too so it's brilliant that you're wearing it.

I have a lovely rose quartz mala given to me by Swamiji when my parents died, and this was an extremely intimate and vital part of the pink ensemble. I was never far away from it during my trips to hospital. Judy was at that time working on her *Crystal Oracle* cards and was having fun pulling them out on my behalf. She sent this:

Anandalite™: cosmic consciousness

Iridescent Anandalite reminds us that consciousness is omniscient and ominpresent, seeing all, knowing all, and that we create our world. Immerse yourself in a quantum field, the holographic universe, and the mystical inter-connectedness that is cosmic consciousness.

Vibration: exceptionally high
Chakra: Higher crown. Cleanses and actives all
Timing: present moment
Soul path: becoming a vessel for cosmic consciousness

Self-understanding: You have the potential to live in a completely different dimension of consciousness. Recognise that you previously operated within a very narrow band of awareness. Attune to flashes of divine light within your soul to take you into the interconnectedness of life. Let feelings of separation fall away and embrace unity. Anandalite gently facilitates integration and releases emotional blockages standing in the way of spiritual awakening.

Divination: You are here to experience cosmic consciousness. Transform your goals and seek a new direction. You have exceptionally clear sight at this time. You find yourself stripped to the bone as the old falls away, do not despair, new light is infused. Know that when you transform your awareness, humanity experiences a quantum shift.

Healing insight: Enlightenment can happen right now. You are part of everything and everything is part of you.

Wow. That was pretty accurate. I was certainly being destroyed from the inside out by the chemo and as we know, nature abhors a vacuum. I was being given space and time for introspection; I was also wondering just how I was going to get through all this and who and how I would be at the end of it all. But we can never know the outcome when we start on a major – and forced – journey like this. Something I still struggle with is the concept of one-ness and everybody being part of the whole. It makes sense to me that we are all connected – so the rose isn't just a rose etc., but it doesn't give a lot of support in facing the fear of a life-threatening illness, or the horrible side effects from the treatment. At those times I was very much on my own. Nobody else could get in my head and comfort me or do it for me – so I felt anything but connected to the greater consciousness. I felt like shouting out "No, we are not all one, because I'm having to go through all this and you aren't." Where's the Oneness and fairness in that?

No answer to that, obviously.

My deep thoughts were often punctuated by wonderful people like the lovely and effervescent Barnaby Roberts who used to work for me at The Wessex Astrologer. We worked together every day for four years and were incredibly close. He was my protégé and I the willing audience to his total nuttiness and deep sensitivity. The day he left to grace another company with his presence was extremely hard, but we have stayed in touch through the years. I was torn apart inside when I had to tell him about the diagnosis – it is so hard to hear somebody being upset on your behalf. But Barnaby was the catalyst that started the whole blog thing off and I am deeply grateful to him for that not very small act. He was upset because he hadn't been included in the loop at one point in the early days, and I was recounting this to Darrelyn when she suggested writing the blog. Barnaby knew that I had always wanted to write and this was the perfect vehicle. He isn't so bad with words himself as shown by his post after blog #7:

Loving this, always knew you would be a superb writer.

Life has given you lemons and you are making pomegranate juice Stephen must have been given grapes at some point which means when you have finished all your nourishing drink, there will be plenty of wine for your book launch.

Can't wait to read this again in its full glory and see what you choose as cover art.

"Wine is constant proof that God loves us and wants to see us happy." – Benjamin Franklin.

What a treasure. However, back to the humdrum existence of a chemo regime, where things were starting to go downhill.

Magic Roundabout

Blog #8 27th January, 2013

I feel duty bound to let you know how things are today, lest you think that so far this has all been exciting hospital visits filled with side-splitting encounters with Dot and the WRVS lady. Make no mistake, today is Horrible. I think a little bit of background is needed here, as to be fair, and somewhat surprisingly, I don't think the chemo is completely to blame. Yes, it has completely toxified my system and definitely debilitated me, but that is what it is supposed to do: as Swamiji said, it is supposed to take my cells to the very point of death so that, like the Phoenix rising from the ashes, my cells can regrow in a more perfect form ready to be zapped by the next lot of chemo. Lovely, I know, but that is how it is, and how it is supposed to be, so I'm not moaning about that.

When I went for the blood tests on Wednesday I mentioned that I felt very fluey and my ears and throat were very sore. Knowing that I need to be as fit and well as possible for the next chemo cycle on 7th February, I wasn't surprised when they prescribed antibiotics. I would normally avoid antibiotics like the plague but my usual measures haven't been working for some months so I thought this would be a good idea. It was a good idea from the point of view of my throat, but taking 500mg of Amoxycillin is never going to help one's intestinal flora – of which there is precious little left after the chemo anyway. Two days of extreme sickness et al followed, so I cut it back by half. First day was better, then yesterday and last night was horrible. But my throat is nearly better (from being sore, obviously not the cancer yet) and that is the bigger picture, so I thought I should be able to cope with a little sickness.

I realise that same picture is becoming complicated and a bit darker than my usual blogs but you are here for the good and the bad, right? I have had a problem with an irregular heartbeat for quite a few years now and although I know it isn't going to kill me, it is incredibly unpleasant when it kicks off as it often lasts for about 36 hours and is completely debilitating. It did so when I was in hospital ready to start chemotherapy, so suddenly all the bedside manner changed from arranging drips and signing consent forms to a lady wiring me up with an ECG trace and the chemo was halted until they had a decision on my heart. I found out a while ago that someone who had a similar problem to me had had an ablation. The electrical circuit of the heart can be upset by cells in one part misfiring and by cauterising those few cells, regular heartbeat can be permanently restored. "Wow, what a brilliant idea," I thought. I'd love one of those. it would solve all my problems.

Fast forward back to lovely Ward 11, drips poised. I kicked my heels for the whole day waiting to see the cardiologist who, very sweetly, was coming after his clinic. That day was quite fun though, as I watched a succession of student nurses tried to complete their regular 'obs' which are blood pressure, oxygen levels and temperature. One of the problems with the irregular heartbeat is that you can't get a true BP reading and of course the heart rate on the oxygen monitor is all over the shop. The NHS is a fabulous institution and has proved itself to be incredible for me, but they don't do a lot of communicating with each other. Student fails to get heart rate, panics after trying both arms, I make sick vampire jokes about bloodletting through my lines and having no heartbeat, student dashes off to get senior person, who hasn't seen the doctor who has ordered the ECG trace. She also can't get BP so she goes to find the other duty doctor who is really lovely but hasn't spoken to the other doctor either so he orders ECG to see what is going on. I say (not for the first time I promise you) that I have already had the trace and I'm waiting to see the cardiologist Later That Same Day. Back down to Defcon 1 and everybody breathes again. Until the next obs check with a new student nurse. Oh no. It did make the time pass quickly though and I got a lot of fun and a lot of mileage out of the vampire scenario.

Will Carling look-alike cardiologist arrives about 5.30. Jolly nice guy, says I have an atrial flutter that won't kill me (that's a relief, just got to beat the cancer then!), and that what I really need is an ablation, but, he looks deep into my eyes and says "I think you know where I am going with this..." Yep, too right, I thought. I would absolutely love a hot wire poked into my heart right now as it is jumping away like a freestyle bungee jumper, but possibly the very aggressive cancer still racing around my system as I haven't started chemo yet is a tiddly bit more important right now. So we mutually agree to try to zap it with a different drug from the one I'm currently on which clearly isn't working. We negotiate the dosage (I lose) and all is set for chemo and a different tablet for my heart the next day. In the event it calmed down as it usually does after a while, so of course they were delighted that the tablet worked. It so didn't. So – anyway, I can have an ablation when I get through 5 months of chemo and a stem cell transplant. Yay! Be careful what you wish for, I say!

Coming slap up to date I woke up this morning with my heart exploding out of my chest. Yes, the drugs don't work.

Apparently the vegas nerve, apart from being responsible for regulating the heart rhythm also regulates the amount of acid in the stomach. Whenever I get the heart problem I also feel really sick from the extra acid that gets released, and dizzy because in beating irregularly you get episodes of several seconds when there is no heartbeat.

Bet you wonder how I ever get any work done :-).

Oh joy. So I don't know whether the heart problem on top of the antibiotic reaction on top of the 6 tablets I have to take every day (plus the injection to boost cell growth) on top of the chemo is making it all extra bad, but I do know that is it now 3.15pm, and the only way I can stay upright is by remaining seated and it is getting incredibly boring. As soon as I move it all goes fuzzy and I feel horribly sick. Which is why I decided the moment had come to share with you, as at least it makes me laugh a bit while I am writing.

The lovely people on Ward 11 said to call them with ANY worry whatsoever, but if I do so I will be on the ward and wired up to something noxious before you know it and I DO NOT WANT MORE DRUGS! Not just yet, anyway. I am dutifully following my yoga breathing and have been clutching rose quartz, speaking gently to my heart and swallowing a lot of chamomile tea. None of which has really made a difference in the past as my heart seems to return to its own rhythm when it is good and ready and not a moment before. But I have to say I am sneaking the ablation threat into my meditations. I'm only human, and you can only be so nice and so calm for so long. When it feels this bad, having a general anaesthetic so I can have a burning wire plunged into my heart seems an incredibly attractive option.

So that is it, you are free to go. I am in excellent hands here as Stephen is looking after me as only a Virgo can and my every need is catered for. Oh yes. Why did I call it Magic Roundabout? Because although I feel I am going in circles and it will be a very long time before I get better, I will indeed get better. And that is pure Magic.

Margaret xx

Times like these were incredibly depressing. I'm not usually a 'poor me' type of person, but it seemed so unfair that I was facing the fight with cancer whilst being knocked sideways by the heart problem. There were many, many tears during this period. I have always (I think!) tried to rise above pain and discomfort by getting involved in my work, or reading, but being this ill meant I really couldn't.

Thank heavens for our two lovely cats, who used to come and keep me company when I was marooned in bed. And you know what it is like with stuff like this... determined to make it to the bathroom on my own without support and end up in tears because I can't. Recover from that episode. A few hours later, must be feeling better enough now to make it to the bathroom without support... fail and cry. It is exhausting and depressing. At those dark times I felt I didn't have the courage of the energy to face all this, and it was only Stephen's gentle and persistent love that kept me going and kept me positive.

Within a few days, and in time for my next appointment, my heart returned to normal. I may not have realized it at the time, but the whole period of treatment would be full of such moments – feeling reasonably well, and then plunging into the depths because things suddenly took a turn for the worse. Something was awakening though, deep inside – which didn't escape Judy's notice, as she sent me this after blog #8:

I know you find Rumi illuminating and I thought this pretty much summed up where you were right now:

> *The breeze at dawn has secrets to tell you. Don't go back to sleep.*
> *You must ask for what you really want. Don't go back to sleep.*
> *People are going back and forth across the doorsill where the two*
> *worlds touch.*
> *The door is round and open. Don't go back to sleep.*

People were indeed going back and forth between worlds on my behalf and there was no way I would be able to go 'back to sleep', or in other words, go back to how I used to be.

The healing circle had kicked in with enormous power coming from many different sources. When I meditate I usually take myself up to a quiet space behind the third eye. I tried this once the healing circle was under way and it nearly blew my socks off. Far from being a quiet place to rest and regroup, it felt as if I was stepping into the Jet Stream. Heady stuff, but the first time nearly reduced me to tears with the sheer wonder of it. So many people tuning in to send me healing.

Wow.

I have been part of many healing circles and groups through the years, but never on the receiving end of it like this. And what stunned me is that several participants told me they sensed who was there, without even knowing by name who was involved. Some key players were kind of 'holding the matrix' including Judy, to make sure that I wasn't overwhelmed. Much like having a room full of highly scented flowers, a massive boost of energy can be a bit hard for a debilitated body to cope with. I found that if I missed the 9.00pm slot due to medical interventions, the energy was there waiting for me at any time. This came in especially useful in the long hours of the long days in isolation after the stem cell transplant, when I was feeling especially bad. Judy was providing on the spot but at a distance support, as she regularly tuned in to check me over on an energetic level and bring messages of support from different entities, as well as my parents, who passed over in 1993.

Working in the Mind, Body, Spirit area of publishing, I am surrounded by different theories on why we are here, and how best to deal with 'life' in all its many-splendoured wonders. What work we still have to do both on ourselves and with others before we leave. This disease was certainly giving me ample material with which to test out different philosophies to how they sat with me. The next blog brought forth a whole lot of such musings.

Dive Deeply into the Miracle of Life

Blog #9 31st January, 2013

Dive deeply into the miracle of life
and let the tips of your wings be burnt by the flame,
let your feet be lacerated by the thorns,
let your heart be stirred by human emotion,
and let your soul be lifted beyond the earth.
Pir Vilayat Inayat Khan Call of the Dervish
(With thanks to Judy Hall for bringing him to my attention)

Quick update on the physical stuff before we move on – my blood count is through the roof, apparently better than a lot of 'healthy' people which is excellent news.

This is of course all to do with the cell-boosting injections and nothing whatsoever to do with all the wheatgrass protein, Vitamin A, Vitamin D3, Flaxseed oil, Whey protein isolate, pomegranate and vegetable juices I have been pouring down my throat, and the stupendous amount of healing that is being sent to me.

It is such a shame that key people within the NHS seem unable to embrace anything that isn't included in a scientific study. If I hear the phrase 'science doesn't support it' one more time I am really going to be tempted... Anyway, I'm free to contemplate my navel for another week then I'm in next Thursday for at least 4 days for Cycle 2, which should be plenty of time to catch you all up on Dot, who gave me a big cheery smile yesterday when I told her I was back in next week. Bless her.

And contemplating my navel is exactly what I have already been doing for several days, starting properly with last Sunday which was definitely the worst day so far. I have been exchanging emails with my dear friend Judy Hall on a wide range of subjects whose common link was the ability to accept, or otherwise, what is going on at the moment, and at her suggestion I'm bringing some of them into the blog so I can think them through in public. I know that sounds weird, but it really helps me – it really is cathartic so thank you for bearing with me.

There are several conflicting trains of thought going on in my head:

1. Interlife planning – Stephen and I planned all this before this reincarnation so that I/we could have a particular experience.

2. Acceptance or surrender to the illness and whatever it is going to teach me/us.

3. Cosmic Ordering. I somehow created this and so with a bit of positive thinking I can get myself out of it.

I fully embrace the belief that we have been here before, and that when we come back we do so to gain particular experiences. Anyone who has read Judy's lovely books The Soulmate Myth *and* The Book of Why *will know from mine and Stephen's story that we feel we have been together for many lifetimes, along with many other case histories in the books. What I struggle to understand is why, in a life that has already included more than its fair share of death and grief I apparently thought it would be a good idea to experience a life-threatening illness, just when things seemed to be going well.*

The whole concept of life after death is usually one that comforts me, but I feel positively grumpy (in my darker moments) that I now have to summon the energy to deal with this massive thing that has come crashing into our lives. I was looking forward to sunny cruises of increasing length, driving in a casual fashion most of the way around the UK to see all the places we have never visited, nice stuff like that. Before you all scream at me that I still can, and that I need to have positive goals for after I am better, yes I know all that. And I do. But in the darkest hours before dawn there's a part of me that is like a petulant and very upset child, shouting 'BUT I DON'T WANT TO DO THE BIT IN-BETWEEN!' And looking forward to a lovely holiday has a completely different feel to it when you insert 5 months of unpleasant treatment in front of it, trust me.

But I have no choice, as I have said before, I can't just call Ward 11 and say that I'm not going to play any more. 'Um, Hi, yes it's Margaret Cahill. This is just to let you know I'm not taking you up on your offer of treatment after all because it is really going to make me feel awful.' Well I could, but that would be stupid in the extreme. It is hard enough to get into remission with this cancer even with the treatment so there is no way I am refusing it. I have no doubt that the reason for having to go through all this will become obvious to me – and this does in fact give me comfort, although it doesn't appear so from the above. To feel that I am treading a path that has spiritual intention gives me focus and a feeling that I am not alone. Someone, some-where presumably has the original plan...

Which brings me on to acceptance, which is a word I think is bandied around far too lightly. It is a very simple word with a huge amount of clout behind it. Accepting seems to me to be a very passive state, which doesn't sit at all well with my cardinality. Taking what comes with non-judgement, being at peace with events beyond your control, staying calm and focussed in the face of adversity. Loving kindness. It all sounds totally brilliant un-til you are faced with a non-negotiable situation, then you realise that to survive this you HAVE to accept it. So acceptance isn't a voluntary deci-sion, it is a coping mechanism that the majority of us probably haven't had to use very much. It is submission on a grand scale to forces way beyond our control, as a means of staying sane. That is the bit that gives my in-ner child the grief, which is on its own something to explore... Hmmm.

When I think about surrender it reminds me of a conversation I had many years ago with Swamiji. I was asking for her help with a mantra that I wanted to use to help me meditate – a little phrase that I could use to give my brain something to do to keep it out of mischief. I was working on something to do with giving everything that I was/am/will be back to God – to become an empty vessel that could wait quietly for direction. She pointed out that whatever it was I thought I was giving back wasn't actually mine to give in the first place – what we agreed on, and what felt right, was that I was surrendering everything willingly, and it is a concept that has drawn me ever since. There is something that works for me in the act of surrendering that doesn't, yet, in acceptance. Acceptance brings out the sulky, 'No don't want to', inner child, whereas surrendering is still difficult but somehow I feel am being allowed to make that decision myself. As you can see, I still have a long way to go with this, and the idea of surrendering to the cancer sounds weird. I can theoretically accept cancer but I can't surrender to it as that has connotations of giving up. I can, however surrender my current situation and give up the idea that I have any power over its outcome. That little sentence is going to provoke a few comments!

Which brings me nicely to the idea of Cosmic Ordering. I would like to say, first off, that many decades ago I was involved for a (very) short time with Amway. Now everybody knows about network marketing and how bad it is, blah, blah, blah, so we're not going down that route at all. What I do want to point out is that their personal development programmes were second to none, and through them I was introduced to the power of Positive Thinking. For that I am very grateful.

This was a Very Long Time before the New Age movement hijacked it and cosmic ordering became the buzzword for having a successful life. I would say that having a positive attitude is incredibly important and I would like to think that I am usually in possession of one (Dark Nights of the Soul excepted), and that it has indeed helped me through some very difficult times. My mother used creative visualisation to help her survive breast cancer for much longer than expected – without any treatment whatsoever – and it figures very strongly in my own meditations. Something has to give the chemo soldiers direction!

I think the danger with taking this concept too far is that it is very obvious if you fail, which is a very heavy burden especially with illness, and for the person who is sick. Quite apart from the shock of an unpleasant diagnosis it is almost too much to take on board that I could have caused this because my thinking was wrong. If we all had our thinking straight everyone would live forever. Nobody lives forever, so excuse me, but isn't there an obvious flaw here?

How can we be vigilant on all fronts so nothing bad sneaks in? And how can we continually programme our thoughts so they only bring good?

We can't.

Let me give you an example of how this can go very wrong, and how you can actually start worrying what you think about. A while ago I heard a rich rock star saying that the best thing about having money was that he was able to put his family through regular MRI scans – a potential problem had already been picked up and he was incredibly grateful to have had that early warning. Great idea, I thought. I added that to my list too. First thing I had after the diagnosis was an MRI scan. I have long wanted to write but never had a subject and certainly never had the time. Look at me now.

Working part time with long periods of enforced seclusion due to treatment. Lots of time to write. I could go on, but I am sure you can see where I am headed. I shared this (and many other very recent examples of 'be careful what you wish for') with Swamiji as I was genuinely starting to worry that I was indeed creating my own reality in completely the wrong way. She has these wise words:

... In the Yoga Vasishtha the great sage Vasishtha tells his disciple Rama in no uncertain terms 'whether enlightened or still in darkness, our own mortality sets fear in us'. One of the ways the New Age movement masks this fear is with the belief that if we can just get our thinking right we will be able to get everything right – transcend our illnesses, our failures, our difficulties. In other words, we have a means of control. And if we don't transcend these things it's not this theory that's wrong, but rather we hadn't got our thinking 'right'. This does seem to me very much like blaming the victim. Life is full of challenges and no matter how 'right' we think, we WILL lose some of these battles, and at our end, we lose the fight we make for life. Not because we got something wrong but because that is the nature of life itself. Not that we have no responsibility. Indeed, we must get our thinking right. We must get our diet, our exercise, our attitude – right. And we must fight every day to do this knowing that we may win the battle today, but we will definitely lose it tomorrow...

So there we have it. To someone who will only see blessings not problems, or who is accustomed to 'ordering' what they want the universe to bring them, this is probably an absolute travesty, but I find it quite helpful. In a perverse way I am almost enjoying the opportunity to plumb the depths of my soul. I am equally sure that both for Stephen and me there are hidden gifts along this difficult path if we only have the courage to seek them out. I leave you with something more from Pir Vilayat Inayat Khan:

> *There is a need to dance the cosmic joy of Shiva. Yet we seem to have cut the possibility of doing it out of our lives and to have fed ourselves with ersatz pleasures. We sacrifice joy for pleasure and try to entertain ourselves with very puny things indeed – things that are really very soul-killing. The real breakthrough of joy only happens when we are moved to the core of our being – when we are shattered by our encounter with meaningfulness.*

Thank you for sharing this time with me. Be well.
Margaret xx

This blog in particular attracted some interesting comments as people welcomed the opportunity to talk about how we find our way through these life-threatening situations. Judy posted this:

Dearest Margaret – this has kind of turned into a blog entry of its own but I thought people who hadn't explored the idea of soul plans might find it thought provoking.

You mention The Book of Why *and I have very fond memories of working on that book with you, the perceptive questions you asked and the insights you willingly offered up. You made me think. Just as your blog does now. I've been exploring people's soul plans – as well as their karma, which is different – for over forty-five years and from our earthly perspective I don't think we can ever know the whole breadth of 'Why'. But of one thing I'm sure, this cancer is part of your soul plan not your karma. It is a means of growing your soul. One of the most important parts of growing your soul seems to be the compassionate witnessing of your own journey and that of others. That's an opportunity you are giving those of us who read your words – and we'll be less judgemental of the journey of another person because of it as you share your insights gained along the way. You are giving all of us who read your words an invaluable gift – and an insight into what you and your higher self – and Stephen – planned for this incarnation.*

I laughed when I reread Margaret Koolman's words that I'd quoted to end The Book of Why: *"when we are coming from the small self, we are like children rebelling against parents." I'm sure you'll resonate with that! She suggests that "to shift what might be going on, you might like to try just sitting with the situation quietly accepting how it is – Saturn delivers the facts, it doesn't require that you judge them or yourself. From that quiet place, choose what you will do, taking care not to judge your choice – just agree with yourself to follow through in order to experience the results of that. To be able to make a choice and follow through IS freedom." She was writing about the Saturn-Uranus opposition but it works just as well for higher-self v. small-self issues and it helps to find dynamic acceptance as well as surrender. To me, this is the point of soul evolution. This experience is giving you incredible soul growth. One thing is for sure, you'll never again feel abandoned, for instance, not with 17,000 hits and counting on your blog! This seems appropriate to remind you of too:*

Now is there civil war within the soul:
Resolve is thrust from off the sacred throne
By clamorous Needs, and Pride the grand-vizier
Makes humble compact, plays the supple part
Of envoy and deft-tongued apologist
For hungry rebels.
Our deeds still travel with us from afar,
And what we have been makes us what we are.
Full souls are double mirrors, making still
An endless vista of fair things before,
Repeating things behind.
Hath she her faults? I would you had them too.
They are the fruity must of soundest wine;
Or say, they are regenerating fire
Such as hath turned the dense black element
Into a crystal pathway for the sun.
　　　　(George Eliot, **Middlemarch***)*

You are amazing, a truly beautiful soul that is being polished to perfection on your crystal road to the sun.
Big hugs
xxJ

Gulp. It was, and still is, very hard to accept the lovely things people say. It isn't until we are in the most life-threatening situations that we think of saying these things. Very humbling indeed.

Acceptance versus surrender was a popular theme, and not one that we usually have to consider in everyday life. Sue had this to say:

Very interested in your thoughts about acceptance, and surrender I was suddenly reminded of a lecture attended by Beau [Sue's son] and I, given by Eva Schloss, Anne Frank's childhood friend, who was with her in Auschwitz. No pontification here. I shall quote Eva's words. We were seated in the front row directly below Eva's lectern. During questions from the floor, Beau, passionately moved by the story of Anne Frank asked "How did YOU keep going? How did you manage to survive?"

"Well," said Eva leaning over her lectern to look at him directly, "I can tell you. It wasn't about bodies. We had no bodies. It was all about mind. My mother said that we must never give up and we didn't!"

I have always thought that was inspirational but reading your blog it occurs to me that energy, help beyond self, and timing also have their parts to play. You still have the mental energy, You are receiving help beyond your self, and despite the chaos that periodically crops up, the timing is working for you. Acceptance and Surrender surely can't be words for you for now.

Then the next day, after more thought, she added:

Even before I begin reading your No 9 again, I can already see how I was wrong, in that acceptance of and 'surrendering to' might ease your return journey to wellness. Interestingly I wasn't happy with 'surrendering' – I wanted the word 'tolerating', and had to keep fighting it off.

To tolerate' is fundamentally pro-active, not a passive apology for a verb like 'to surrender' – so that's my bête noir then. God keep me from experiencing at first hand the strength of surrendering – but he won't keep me from it will he? See what your inside-out-sharing does for your readers?

It's good to get everyone going! It was also nice to get comments back and to realize that nobody else has the answer either. I was beginning to see that the only thing all these different philosophies can offer us is a coping strategy to help us through difficult times. One person's acceptance is someone else's surrender. Interesting. Still not convinced by Cosmic Ordering though. Much as it was so horribly difficult going through all this, a part of my soul was kind of reaching out and sighing into the space that was being granted for a lot more inner delving. In the midst of our busy lives it is very seldom that we have the opportunity for much navel contemplation. I now had it in spades, which was surely a gift, but not one I planned putting in the supermarket trolley of Life. My progress in the acceptance and surrender department was brought to the fore the very next day.

Hair Today, Gone Tomorrow

Blog #10 1st February, 2013

*The day has finally arrived. After much inner deliberating and outer brav-
ery we finally shaved my head today. But of course there is a story I have to
share with you, one to really gladden the spirit.*

*My first thought after 'Oh no, lymphoma means it is cancer' was 'Oh
no, I'm going to lose my hair.' My younger son Matt has said in the past
that my hair defines me – usually when I have been moaning about its total
madness and inability to look good when I need it to. There was lots and lots
of it and everyone loved it except me. I longed for straight, glossy, swishy
hair like they have in the adverts, but I was in the curly queue when the hair
quota was given out. Shortly after that I joined the very end of the patience
queue, and they ran out before I got to the front, but that's a whole other
story.*

*Several people had suggested that I shave my head before the actual event
as a mark of control in a situation where, for the most part, I have no control
at all. I completely agreed but decided to wait until my hair showed signs
of departing from my head of its own accord, simply because I had heard of
people who had this treatment and didn't lose their hair. And I was convinced that I was going to be a medical miracle and not lose mine too.*

*Everything in cancer treatment has a day number, as chemo treatment
begins on Day 1. Obviously. It is a number that must be recited to whichever medical person asks. Failure to recite your day number elicits a look of
total disbelief that you can be so out of touch with your treatment.*

*One of the very first questions I asked was when I'd lose my hair, and
I was told between days 10 and 14. Chemotherapy really is such a precise
science – they know exactly when things are going to happen – it's really
quite amazing.*

*So at Day 10, I gave my hair a good tug and it was really well attached.
At Day 11, I actually had a compliment that my hair was looking really
nice, so that was a result. Days 12 and 13 were similarly good and I was
thinking, 'YES! Beaten the system! One more day to go!' Day 14 arrived.
The tug on my hair was only half-hearted as I knew by now that I Would
Be Different. At the half-hearted tug a whole clump of hair came away in*

my hands. How cruel is life? I was right up in front of the finishing post, so close to hairy victory, when at the last moment it was snatched from my grasp. Literally. So for a couple of days I kept checking it was still falling out, with the result that, well, it kept falling out. Shaving it should have been really easy. I knew it was the sensible thing to do for loads of reasons and mostly because it should have felt like I was in control. But it didn't. I was really grieving for the old me and knew this would be the final step I had to take to move fully into the future.

I delayed for a couple of days, then this morning what was left looked so awful, and the scarves I had bought felt so uncomfortable that I said to Stephen, "Let's just do it." We dillied and dallied, fed the cats, washed up from last night, dithered around, then finally I sat down so he could apply the clippers. It felt really weird. Then, when he was halfway across my head, the doorbell rang.

It was the postman with a big brown box. Our lovely friends Jack and Kris, from the American Federation of Astrologers in Arizona, had said they were preparing a mystery present for me and this was it. Trailing bits of hair across the floor, I was desperate to see what it might contain – only without opening it – it is so much more fun that way and prolongs the excitement. I saw the green customs label and saw that it contained... hats.

As an astrologer I know that timing is everything, but how stunningly appropriate was that? Sadness turned to excitement and I couldn't wait for my hair to be finished so I could look in the box. I was stunned. The box was filled with beautiful, handknitted hats. And they were all pink.

Unbeknown to me, Jack's sister Carol makes hats as a part time hobby and he had ordered loads to come to me. They are totally individual and real works of art. I shall model them and put them up for you to see one by one as she deserves to sell as many as she can possibly make. Her website is hatsbycarol.com. She transformed my day with her artistry as did Jack and Kris by their love and caring. Thank you all, from the bottom of my heart. Happy Friday!

So that was it. I was a fully paid up member of the cancer club, immediately identifiable wherever I went. The hats were amazing, and a real talking point once I got used to the idea. I was having severe hot sweats due to the menopause, so we had already decided not to lash out on an expensive scratchy wig. Can you imagine how mad it would look, being out in public and whipping my hair off in the midst of soaring body temperatures? Not that I took my hat off in public, but at least I could lift the edges to let some air in when the need arose.

Losing my hair also gave rise to a whole new load of jokes. You don't realize how many times little sayings come out: "I take my hat off to you", "Keep your hair on", "that's really splitting hairs", which all become really funny in a sick kind of way. I gained a huge amount of sympathy for Stephen, who started losing his hair in his twenties and now wears what is left very short. Hats both to keep warm and provide shade from the sun have become a necessary part of the wardrobe.

Going out the first few times was really awkward. We bumped into a neighbour that we hadn't seen for a long time (clearly!) and she commented that I was looking very demure. I was wearing a headscarf at the time so could quite possibly have looked as if I had joined a sect where women keep their heads covered. So of course I had to tell her... which led to a great long conversation but again a lot of support. I hated being immediately identifiable; dealing with this cancer was supposed to be a private thing – except for the blogs but nobody could see me on there – and now I felt like I was wearing a big badge proclaiming my membership to the cancer club. It is horrible having to deal with this very obvious manifestation of the treatment whilst still coming to terms with the havoc it causes body mind and spirit.

Once I got into the cycle of chemo treatments there was almost a security in knowing I was going in for treatment again to beat this thing. I was feeling well enough to go into work on some days, or at least work from home, but it was a very disjointed existence as there was always at least one hospital visit a week and after discharge the daily visits from the nurse. I was planning hard for the next visit as I knew it would be longer and more arduous and I wanted to get through it in the best possible shape.

Countdown to Cycle Two

Blog #11 5th February, 2013

Just 2 days to go until I'm back in hospital to start Cycle 2, and I'm beginning to feel like an old-timer :-). At least I know what to take in with me now as having your own things around you really helps. It sounds a bit like the game I used to play with my sons, I went on a Picnic and I Took....So this is, I Went into Hospital and I Took: a duvet in a bright pink cover (they really don't have blankets, more like thick sheets which don't keep you warm), my own (pink) towels (theirs are horrible and scratchy), my own mug – pink, obviously (no more negotiations about tiny green cup or tiny white mug for me!), apples (they aren't big on fruit in there), tea bags (herbal tea also isn't on the menu), black and pink cat slippers (a present from Stephen and they make everyone chuckle which is lovely), and obvious things like the iPod, Kindle, proper books and laptop. I'd really love to take the cafetière too but apart from the fact I'm probably not allowed near a kettle for health and safety reasons, there is a real danger I'd end up competing with The Tea Trolley and that would be a Really Bad Thing. In short I need a train of Sherpas following me into the ward, but it has to be done.

And clothes. I like to get up and dressed every day as I don't feel I represent myself very well when clad in fluffy pyjamas (usually pink) and you never know when you might have to have a serious conversation with the consultant. Honestly though, things like that do matter. It is really hard to fully participate in a ward round with a whole bunch of medical people around your bed and retain any sense of posture when they are in day clothes and you aren't. Especially as I want to talk to them about drug trials.

Although the staff get you to sign consent forms and tell you all about the treatment you will be having and encourage you to ask questions, they don't REALLY want you to ask big questions like, do I really have to take this? Or anything that veers away from the straight and narrow. The understanding is very much that they have the answers and you go in there to be treated and not ask serious questions.

I don't deny for a moment that they most probably do have the answers and I am reliant on them to get well. However, I do need to be asking some questions. It seems there are two new drugs being trialled in the US and Germany which are proving to be effective, and with a lot less toxicity. At the moment they are only being used on people who have relapsed after a complete cycle of chemo and for whom it won't work a second time. I can understand those patients being a priority, but I would also like to see whether I can get my name put forward if there are trials on new cases.

I mentioned a few blogs back that Mantle Cell Lymphoma is on the increase, which from my point of view is good news as more research is being directed at understanding and treating it, and it seems that for the first time there may actually be a cure on the horizon.

Hospital does really weird things to your thought processes and I can see how easy it would be to become institutionalised. As someone said to me, you go in there and are not expected to do anything in return. In fact there isn't anything you can do as it is all set up to look after you and to not expect anything back, even if you are completely able-bodied a lot of the time, like in the cancer ward. That could be quite an attractive short-term proposition if it wasn't for the food.

I jest of course. You could theoretically spend the whole day looking at the wall and nobody would do much to stop you, which is incredibly bad for the spirit, especially as the hospital got massive discount on that really dreary cream colour. We are allowed to drag our drips around even as far as the shop, so I might do that just for a change of scenery and for a laugh at some point, although I do take a lot of things in to help keep boredom at bay.

Something I am really enjoying is Zentangle. Have you heard of it? Stephen had a review copy of a Zentangle book come into the office and I was immediately hooked. I really am not in the slightest bit artistic. Even my stick men don't look like stick men and pre-school children can turn out far better paintings than I. This has always frustrated me as the yearning was there but the talent clearly wasn't. Look it up – it is meditation and art in partnership. It is in fact the kind of doodles we all did at school except with a posh name and a whole lot of marketing and money behind it – but one little book and you are away. I'll put one of mine up when I can take a decent picture. But I have to say you can get lost in it for hours, which is a very useful thing for hospital stays, and it really does free your mind. You build it up one tiny section at a time with the end result being something really quite impressive. Then you look at it and think 'Wow, I really can draw!'. Of course I still can't draw, but it looks nice and it is very good for the soul.

I did of course miss something off the list – hats. Readers of the last blog will realise I now have a splendid selection of headwear to choose from, which is just as well as my head really does get cold now. I didn't realise how much my hair was keeping me warm! I've had a few days now of decreasing coverage – once we shaved it all off it was easier to manage, but even the tiny little bits are falling out now and soon I will be as bald and shiny as an archetypal little alien. Not a teeny hair in sight. So I will need hats in hospital.

Judy came to see us on Saturday and as well as bringing a ton of pomegranates and dragon fruit (more of that in a moment) she also took photos of me and Stephen in a couple of the hats – Stephen was game enough to wear a fetching black and pink number. I know it is important for partners to be supportive but I think he excelled himself on this occasion!

Dragon fruit, known also as Pitaya, is apparently packed with antioxidants and Vitamin C and the tiny seeds are rich in Omega 3. It tastes a bit like kiwi fruit but it is a lot more exciting to look at. The outside is brilliantly red and exotic, while the inside resembles weird grey-fleckled polystyrene. Would certainly get the conversation going around the dining room table! Many thanks to Morrisons and Judy for supplying us with it.

I could also have taken some pictures of the kitchen after we juiced some of the pomegranates. It honestly looked like the Chainsaw Massacre. Those little bits of pomegranate fruit really don't want to come out, and to turn them into juice is truly a labour of love. Michele suggested in a comment on an earlier blog that I embrace the myth of Persephone and her trip to the Underworld as a meditative approach to the process. I think I might need that to stay calm!

So tomorrow I visit the lovely people on Ward 10 for more bloodletting and a pre-admission check then it's all systems go on Thursday. I would imagine I'll be back with a blog around Saturday when the tedium of being attached to a drip is really beginning to wear a bit thin. I'll be sending your regards to Dot :-).

Good night

Margaret xx

A visit from Judy is always exciting. She often brings crystals but always arrives with a wonderful all-embracing energy that allows almost anything to happen – and it usually does. On this occasion, after taking excited pictures of new hats and trying the dragon fruit, we got talking about muscle testing, which I haven't tried for a while. Judy's visit interestingly enough coincided with the arrival of Bob Makransky's shipment of Jorobte leaves. Bob is one of my authors; he lives in Guatemala and had recently sent some suggestions to help treat the lymphoma with earth magic rituals from his *Earth Magic* book which included earth burial. Obviously alive. I was a bit put off by that idea as I can imagine getting really claustrophobic being buried up to my chin in earth – or sand. Just in case anyone out there is braver than me, this is what you do:

> *Another ritual which can be used in conjunction with or apart from the daily earth ritual is the burial ritual. You use this one whenever you are especially burdened, ill, careworn, or depressed. The earth has an infinite capacity not only to heal but also to absorb and dissipate negative energy, and every sort of spiritual and emotional heaviness as well as chronic illness.*
>
> *It helps to fast the day before this ritual. Dig a trench two feet deep and somewhat longer than your body. Line the trench with sawdust or leaves so you will have a soft bed and pillow to lie on, and make sure your face will be shaded from the sun. Disrobe and wrap yourself in a sheet with only your face exposed (the sheet serves as a protection against e.g. ants). You can smear insect repellant on your face, neck, and hair to keep bugs away. Then lie down in the trench, get comfortable, and have someone cover you with a layer of earth up to your neck with your head sticking out. Have someone visit you every hour or two in case you need a drink and to make sure you're okay. If you have to pee, just do it.*
>
> *If you are very sick or in desperate need of lightening up, you should remain buried for 12 hours (dawn to dusk) the first time you bury yourself, and for at least 6 hours on subsequent burials (8 is better). Average people only need four hour burials to tune themselves (there's not much point in doing it for less than four hours at a stretch). How long and how frequently you bury yourself depend*

on how sick or heavy you were to begin with: you come to "know" when it's time to bury yourself again.

Although this ritual may seem to be an odd thing to do, you might just find that being buried is one of the most enjoyable experiences you've ever had. The earth herself is your hostess, and she will do her best to comfort, nourish, and entertain you.

Another way of making intimate contact with the earth is to walk around barefoot as much as possible. If you live in a place where you can't walk around barefoot, maybe it would be worthwhile to move to a place where you can – it is that important. Wearing shoes cuts off most of the healing energy and sense of rootedness which the earth would otherwise give us through our feet.

These rituals aren't immutable – you can alter them at will to suit your own taste and convenience. What is important is your seriousness of purpose, the strength of your desire to communicate with the earth, and your willingness to pursue this intent in a deliberate fashion – to make it one of the high priorities in your life. Then your success is assured: you will find a true sense of worth and belonging in the world which doesn't depend on what other people think of you.

Very thought provoking. We got into earthing and walking barefoot a bit later on, and certainly the feeling was amazing. I hadn't realized how disconnected I was. I am usually quite a chilly person, so walking barefoot is out of the question for most of the year in England, but I am certainly going to make more of an effort to do so in the future.

I did however accept Bob's offer of Jorobte leaves, which I would drink like a tea. I was amazed that the package made it through Customs to be honest, but I was very eager to try it once it had arrived. Eager but slightly apprehensive. I have had a lot of herbs before and they all tasted terrible. A notable example of this was when Swamiji sent over some herbs to me when I was suffering from really bad flu, many years ago. It was dutifully made up for me and it didn't even smell that bad. But the taste was out of this world in a Very Bad Way. And the worst feature of it was the effect it had on my mouth; sucking tree bark is the only comparison that springs to mind even now, several decades later. So – I tried to be brave – but my body rebelled as soon as the liquid hit my mouth. And I was supposed to drink about four cups of this a day. Oh dear.

Back in the energy-testing conversation with Judy, we started out by setting up the control; I held out my right arm to the side and Judy asked me if my name was Margaret Cahill. I said yes, and as I did so she pushed down on my arm, which stayed straight and strong because I was telling the truth. Muscle testing is very strange. It is based on the Chinese system of diagnosis through the meridians, and it can be used to test the usefulness of a potential treatment or medicine.

The idea is to hold the medicine/food/whatever in one hand and raise the other one to the side. The person assisting pushes down on your arm while you ask whether the item/idea/treatment etc. is good for you. If your arm goes down easily the answer is negative.

The funny thing about it is that when it is a negative answer you can't actually do anything to make your arm strong. So when asking if wine was a good thing for me, I found that no amount of strengthening would keep my arm up. I held the dragon fruit and we got a positive answer – my arm didn't move. I held a variety of other pills and potions, and then we asked whether chemo was good for me. We got a surprisingly positive answer. Not that I would have stopped it on the basis of energy testing, but I didn't expect that. Presumably 'good' in the sense that it would annihilate the cancer. That was positive then...

Then I held the Jorobte leaves and we got a very definite 'No'. That surprised me too as it tasted so foul I assumed it would be very good for me and that my body disliking it so violently was only to be expected. Isn't medicine supposed to taste bad?! Talking of bad I wasn't looking forward to telling Bob that I wasn't taking his medicine after he went to the effort of acquiring then sending it.

But that is the difficulty when you are ill; well-meaning people send all kinds of ideas and suggestions for diets, therapies and books, and they aren't all relevant or practical. I really felt quite bad when I rejected an idea... I didn't want to upset the person suggesting it so

I quietly stored them away until I was asked about it, hoping that I wouldn't be. Which of course was another part of my learning process: being brave enough to tell the truth even if it involved possibly upsetting someone.

There is such a lesson here about setting expectations and allowing possibilities. Telling the truth without any 'dangly bits' or hidden agenda, and no expectation of the outcome allows a much purer flow of energy. Childhood experiences of people telling me I couldn't do something (which happened quite a lot as I wanted to do quite a lot of impractical stuff) had set me up to expect negative answers; the reality was that people appreciated being told the truth and it opened the way to much wider discussion and exploration. It is very much a work in progress even now.

At this point Judy was about to go on holiday to Egypt. As an avid and very knowledgeable Egyptologist, she gets into the temples and monuments that others don't, and she went off merrily clutching our photo. Little did I know I was about to get an up-close introduction to Egyptian Deities! Contact between us was obviously limited, but almost immediately she started sending through photos of us placed in temples and on statues. A particularly beautiful one featured Judy holding us in the temple of Philae. Terrie Birch, one of her travelling companions, takes the most surreal photographs – truly a psychic photographer, and this particular one showed a shaft of light going straight down through the photo of us that Judy was holding. On an energetic level it felt amazing to know that I was receiving healing from such high places. I was getting my own personal healing and travel blog, direct from the Sphinx's mouth…

Hi Margaret,

Greetings from Luxor. Your photo in the pink hat went to Karnak yesterday. We'll email you the photo of it sitting on a very large scarab the symbol of the light that becomes 'out of the darkness'. The transforming quality of light. We had to walk 7 times anti-clockwise around the scarab to bring you luck and healing. One other person was walking clockwise – must have been dyspraxic! Good luck for Thursday. Don't forget the feathers!
Hugs and love,
Judy

I commented this back to Judy:

I was thinking of making the next blog about how powerful it is when the sick person is taken around by proxy/photo to places like that; Komilla is having 157,000 pujas chanted for me by a priest in one of the temples she was visiting in India. Feeling supported and cared for across the world is immensely humbling.

And this is the modern day wonder that is the blog. A massive, massive lesson, one that has certainly changed my life since, is that if you open up and let people support you, they will take you to their hearts and their healing will be magnified immensely.

Blood tests and pre-chemo check accomplished, I was ready to take the Sherpa train to Ward 11. Unfortunately I was back in Iso 1, which is the two-bedded room I occupied last time, but without my lovely friend. Freezing cold and very dreary for some reason I can't fathom. Not that any of the rooms are especially wonderful. I was first in so was able to choose my bed – this time I went by the window, which turned out to be the source of the coldness, but at least I had sunlight. Well – daylight!

Cycle Two – As it Happens

Blog #12 9th February, 2013

OK – we are at Saturday morning and the tedium has hit. I came in Thursday and we got cracking on the first round, which was about 3 hours, then for yesterday and today I'm having 2 cycles a day of about 3½ hours each. There is quite a lot of fussing around making everything sterile and checking the dosage so although the actual chemo dose is 3 hours the whole thing takes longer than that. Which isn't so bad if it is all happening in the daytime, but we didn't get started until nearly 10.00 last night so it didn't finish until after 1.00 this morning. Thankfully Stephen had bought me the boxed set of Sex and the City, *so Carrie and the Girls saw me safely through until the bitter end.*

I managed to get settled down and asleep by about 1.30 and was having the most amazing dream. I think wonderful dreams are sent sometimes just to give us a break from the less pleasant things we have to go through – a sort of mental holiday. I was sublimely foxtrotting round a ballroom (and yes, I can foxtrot, and it is my favourite dance) with lovely swing music playing and sort of misty edges to the ballroom so it just faded away. I was probably wearing one of those amazing floaty dresses from Strictly Come Dancing, *but I can't remember now because next it was "GOOD MORNING! HOW ARE YOU TODAY? CAN I JUST TAKE YOUR BLOOD PRESSURE?" and my lovely dream was torn asunder.*

Lights full on, I was dragged kicking and screaming into the reality of Saturday and another day of treatment.

I've decided to stop talking about the treatment being toxic as thinking that way creates such a horrible reaction in my body as it goes in. We all know it is extremely toxic and that it burns skin on contact, but the alternative isn't exactly attractive either so I am concentrating on visualising the chemicals as a force for good sloshing through my veins. (More of the soldiers later.) It does feel quite weird though and you gradually get a horrible taste in your mouth, which is something I learnt from Cycle 1 can be minimised if you have something to eat or suck while the drip is attached. With this in mind we went out last week to find some lozenges.

We headed, somewhat misguidedly as it turns out, for the health food shop, expecting them to have a wider range of additive-free fare. How wrong could we be? I don't understand why the company who manufacture the leading brand of 'healthy' lozenges go to all the trouble of growing herbs organically on a Swiss mountain side then adulterate them with sugar and glucose syrup, or in the sugar-free variety, aspartame.

If you don't know the background of those last two, go look them up. One place they shouldn't be is in food, and I think we can be fairly sure that they aren't there for our benefit. The only thing we found in the entire shop was Real Fruit Snack Bars, which have – just real fruit puree! What a pleasant surprise! They are flat and moist so are kind of doing the job, but if you do come across something suitable I'd love to know.

We are allowed to bring food in, but I already have my big container of fresh juice in the fridge and space is at a premium. It does astound me what the hospital serve up to people who are already ill. Dot offered me yoghurt on my first visit as we searched the menu for sugar and additive free options and she was stunned to find that the 'healthy' fruit yoghurt actually had very little fruit or yoghurt in it – the ingredients were mostly corn syrup, guar gum and flavourings.

It does make me sad that our food is so adulterated nowadays that I imagine a lot of people couldn't actually cope with live, natural yoghurt with a bit of real fruit mixed in – not without dumping a load of sugar in it. I'll just jump off that particular soapbox before it becomes too boring. But do, please, go and read a few labels. It is illuminating reading if nothing else!

I thankfully haven't had much to do with hospitals in the past, and I hadn't realised how much of nursing is the daily grind of handing out medication, changing dressings and checking vital signs. I especially hadn't realised how fascinating and complicated bowel habits are.

Joking aside, these are the first sign of something going wrong with a chemo patient so you wouldn't believe how much detail you have to go into. I take my pink hat off to the fabulous nurses on this particular ward for making these small interactions so much fun, and for really, really caring about doing the best job they can for the patients.

The nice thing about coming back to the same ward is that you get to know everyone. One of the nurses is getting married soon, and last time I was in here she had planned a day out with her mum and the bridesmaids to track down The Dress, but the bad weather was making it all look distinctly dodgy. I am happy to report that the trip was a success. Another nurse had planned a chocolate-themed birthday party for her daughter, and having had a chocolate fountain at our party a few years ago, with disastrous results, I was particularly eager to find out how that went and if they do them for adults :-D. It went really well and no they don't, just so you know.

So, thinking about soldiers and helpful liquid sloshing through my veins, I realise that my attitude and thus my needs are changing. My Mars in Aries has quietened down considerably through this experience and the soldiers don't need to go storming through my system like they did.

This is actually very welcome, as I didn't really feel it was right for me. Even in the beginning, I didn't feel that I was 'fighting' this cancer. I've never done that well with fighting things anyway, and maybe I felt instinctively that I would use all my energy on trying to win the battle and have none left at the end to enjoy life.

The happiest and most inspiring people seem to talk about living with cancer and that makes more sense to me. Cancer is now a part of my life, and the spectre of it in the form of regular tests will always be there; we would have a very uncomfortable existence if it was a continually antagonistic relationship. Fighting also doesn't marry well with the exceptionally beautiful healing I am receiving. In the light of this I am working hard at being kind to myself and my body, as it was the reverse of those conditions that made it sick. To this end I am now seeing the drugs as a positive force gently washing through my system. More thoughts on this theme to follow. I have to admit that today I am a bit bored of the game and want to go home.

The thing I need most is sleep. The first night I was in I was sharing a ward with an older lady who was very uncomfortable and in a lot of pain. Her regular trips to the bathroom were interspersed with periods of snoozing where she was talking in her sleep imploring The Lord to take her. In the wee small hours I had really had enough and went across to ask her if she wanted me to call one of the nurses. To which she replied with a perky "Oh no, love, don't you worry about me, I'm fine!"

Grrr.

So I spent yesterday in a sleep-deprived state and wasn't exactly well-armed to be up until 1.00 on the drip. Today is passing in a bit of a headachey fashion as a side effect of the drugs, but this too shall pass. The end is *in sight and I will have another 3 weeks to recuperate before the next cycle. With my fresh juice lovingly made by Stephen (with NHS straw!) and an almost endless supply of Sex and the City I'm as happy as I could possibly be in the circumstances.*

Have a brilliant weekend.

Margaret xx

I finally got home, under the mistaken impression I would bounce back easily. It wasn't quite as easy as that; I was over-tired and stressed due to the hospital environment (and food, obviously), and my body was starting to react more strongly to the chemo.

I am more than happy with my own company and my natural impulse is to explore within when circumstances without are less than ideal. You can't do that on the ward, so I was really desperate to get out of there. In fact this was the beginning of my strategy to spend as little time in hospital as possible.

I found out that the consultant comes on ward rounds with an expectation which has pretty much been set up by feedback from the nursing staff. Oh yes. Make the gossip machine work for you! I soon realized that by using this crafty tool I could 'influence' the doctor's decision in advance, so that, within reason, their feelings about discharge pretty much matched mine.

Result.

The grass is always greener... But actually it is! I hated being in hospital and my sole mission once admitted was to get out again. I can't understand why people like to stay in for a bit longer, and believe me, they do. They also don't question the system. I was well aware that I was in unknown territory; the nurses knew what to expect after chemo, but I didn't. But ultimately they got to realize that I am pretty sensible and would have called the ward with any worries. That makes it sound like adjusting to coming home and relying on my own intuition was easy, but it wasn't. One very big benefit of being home, however, was being able to experiment with the medication – something that is very hard to do in hospital for obvious reasons.

Inside Out

Blog #13 12th February, 2013

The first few days after I get home from hospital are always very thought provoking. I think we have already established that there is zero opportunity for contemplation on the ward because of the constant interruptions, but also because my body is being subjected to a whole load of trauma; it is only once I get home that I have a chance to find out how it has reacted and what it needs from me to help it recover.

Swamiji gave me some very wise advice before my first treatment: she said I should wait to decide on any supplements and healing until after the treatment and have faith that my body would guide me. It did and it does and it is truly wonderful. Listening to myself is proving to be my way through the maze of debilitation which follows chemotherapy. This cycle was truly horrible, which I understand is a lot to do with the cumulative effect of the treatment – so, mentally, I have to find a way of dealing with this.

Realistically, it will only get worse as I progress through the cycles. I can hear all the positive thinkers amongst you (especially the ones who haven't had chemo) throwing up your hands in horror at such an apparently negative statement, but I think this is really important. I was very lucky to feel comparatively well after the first cycle (antibiotics and palpitations notwithstanding), and I thought I would be equally fine after the second, but that was neither the truth nor a realistic expectation – and the disappointment at the let-down is almost as bad as the feeling bad after the treatment.

Taking Swamiji's advice, and suffering from nausea and headaches, yesterday I retreated within to listen to my body's cries for help. I find it quite easy to get into a meditative state (having had an excellent teacher!) but I was feeling so rough yesterday that I needed something evocative to help get me there. I am totally in love with a video on youtube.com of a flashmob meditation in London on 2nd June 2011 which features the track The End of Suffering, *spoken by Thich Nhat Hanh (with background chanting and music) from the book and CD package* Graceful Passages. *Hopefully you can see it here:*

http://www.youtube.com/watch?v=mqZA5cToPgs. *If not you are all bright enough to go find it for yourselves. The whole flashmob meditation idea really appeals to me and I'd really like to participate in it on a warm sunny day when I am better. Or even if I'm not better – just warm and sunny would be good.*

The rigours of hospital, its lack of peace, extreme bias on western concepts of care (obviously) and awful food take a huge amount out of me, and one is discharged to go home feeling very depleted indeed.

It is pure irony that the doctor always asks, "Do you feel well enough to go home?" I was so close to saying, "No, I feel so bad I have to go home." But didn't.

They have no idea. So I needed the feel good factor, and this video is definitely it. Sunshine, beautiful music, people sitting peacefully in the middle of central London. How much better can it get?

First I watched the clip on youtube then I replayed it, getting myself comfy to just listen to the 7 minute meditation that led me gently into my own, and from where I could tap into the massive stream of healing that has become available to me through all of you lovely people. I was able to let go of the discomfort of my body and soar upwards towards the safe place where I could tune into it and hold it gently as it wept. And weep it did. The chemotherapy is one thing, and I am slowly coming to terms with the necessity of its toxicity, but the other drugs you are given to counteract the side effects are quite another thing as they are unbelievably damaging in their own right. My body was screaming "Noooooooooooooooooo!" to all the other stuff as I meditated. As I came out of the meditation I knew what I had to do.

In hospital I was being given intravenous anti-nausea medication which apparently causes headaches as a side effect. So as well as having the potent anti-emetic I was having paracetamol and codeine to counter the headache. As they weren't lasting the appointed hours before all the discomfort came back I needed other pain relief and other anti-emetics to keep me going… this was getting silly. Especially as there was very little food in my stomach to absorb it. You can see why my body was traumatised.

I used to suffer with migraines as a child, and one of the things I noticed because of that was that the sickness and headache always came back together. Once I got home I thought if I could control the sickness the headache would go. It did. Brilliant! 4 less tablets to take! During the meditation I had discovered this wasn't right either but I didn't know why. I found that the anti-emetic Metaclopromide tablets (different from the one given by IV) were running out before their allotted time.

I wondered about calling the hospital to see whether I could take more, but a little voice in my head said, 'Side effects, Margaret. Look at the side effects'. OMG. I am so pleased I did.

As the drug wore off (often after only 2 hours) I found I just couldn't sit still. I thought it was because of the discomfort from the returning nausea and headache but it is one of the side effects. Once I started reading I was horrified. This is a really seriously heavyweight drug often used in the treatment of migraine (how strange is that? See, my intuition was good!), that has seriously heavyweight side effects – I was thinking of asking to increase it?

I decided to stop taking it and deal with the problem from the headache end first, ably abetted by peppermint tea for the sickness. Hope you aren't bored rigid yet. Anyhow, that sorted out a lot of the problem and I went to bed a much happier and healthier bunny having tipped fewer tablets down my throat.

This morning didn't start well. After such promising progress last night I awoke to my heart exploding out of my chest and the sickness and dizziness I usually get when it does so. Depressed doesn't even begin to cover it. I felt incredibly let down all over again and I couldn't believe that my heart had started to join in with this horrible 3 weekly scenario at exactly the same stage as on the last cycle. I was completely at sea and it was only when a friend arrived to take Stephen out for a (much needed!) coffee that I realised a chance had presented itself to spend some serious 'going within' time. Not that we don't give each other space, it is just different with someone else around. I didn't want to talk, I wanted to ask my body again what it needed.

This disease is providing the most amazing opportunities to seriously experiment with all the various therapies and techniques that have come my way during the last few decades (yes, decades). Although I have had my dark nights in the past, this is definitely the darkest of them all, so a serious road test of several of them is in order.

Several people have mentioned EFT – Emotional Freedom Technique – and I have to say that in the past (and I tried it again when we covered it in Judy Hall's Good Vibrations) it hasn't done a lot for me. I decided to watch a clip of how to do it as sometimes words aren't enough. I found http://www. eft.mercola.com which is an excellent site for a real hands-on, 'how-to' example. I watched it all the way through then repeated it with my own words and let my body guide me. Oh my word. The flood gates opened.

One of our cats, Rowan, was sitting next to me and she made a cat equivalent of 'Ah no, poor you' type of noise and climbed up to lick away my tears. Really.

The only reason I have gone into this much detail is to show people who haven't found time for it, or don't think they need it, HOW IMPORTANT IT IS TO LISTEN TO YOUR BODY. I was drawn to EFT after years of not using it and it provided a massive release for me.

In case you haven't guessed it, I am going through a phase of asking myself what I need – just for those who have done what I do in a slow article and cut to the end to see if it has perked up. Bad habit I inherited from my dear mum. I have had masses of advice from everyone over the last couple of months, and some of it has felt right and some of it I have had to give thanks for and discard. Every approach isn't right for every person. I don't feel like positive self-talk or affirmations (outside of those used in EFT which are different). I have been doing that for years and I am now very ill, so rightly or wrongly, there is something in me that hasn't been recognised in that process and I need to discover what it is. I am using some incredibly powerful books to help me with this:

The Journey *by Brandon Bays*
Broken Open *by Elizabeth Lesser*
Dying To Be Me *by Anita Moorjani*

Fabulous books by fabulous, brave, ladies. I take my pink hat off to them as I delve into the treasures they offer. I run the gauntlet of Ward 10 blood tests tomorrow and all that entails, then some lovely Tibetan Sound Therapy on Thursday, but for the rest of the week I am looking forward to contemplating my navel and seeing what it has to tell me.

This blog might have seemed a bit heavy after the last, but these thoughts need to mature like a good wine... and the periods after chemo seem to be when they do it. And for all those needing to know about drinkies on Sunday night I did ask one of the nurses – it happened to be the one who suggested it on Christmas day, which was a stroke of luck. The bad news was

that the drinks trolley had only offered port and sherry (eeeiuw!) so I wasn't gutted that it hadn't been instigated. I was at home by Sunday anyway and I can assure you that a cool glass of Chardonnay would have ended up a very long way from my stomach at that point :-)
With warm wishes for your ongoing health
Margaret xx

Writing the blog was having a strange effect on me. I had stopped writing in my journal as I felt that the thoughts just sat there and festered. I didn't like that at all. Through the blog I had found a way of connecting with people, sometimes literally from my bed, and I was loving it. I felt as though I was in a constant discussion with them, and it was a huge, huge help as the treatment became more gruelling. Between us Stephen and I know a lot of people, and word had spread fast. Apart from comments on the blog we were both getting loads of emails saying the most wonderful, supportive and lovely things. Opening up like this was quite alien to me, but it was like Pandora's box; my innermost ponderings on the meaning of life now had an outlet, and there was no stopping them.

Weekend Reflections

Blog #14 17th February, 2013

So, I think it is fair to say that I left the last blog in a state of depressed contemplation. Sorry about that :-).

I have to say that on a temporary basis things didn't get better. I woke up in the early hours of Wednesday morning and, thinking my heart had calmed down, tentatively got up to use the bathroom.

It hadn't calmed down.

By the time I had walked the 3 steps to the bedroom door I was dizzy and sick, and came crashing down against the doorjamb, sending the nearby laundry basket flying. Poor Stephen, dragged from his dreams, was with me in seconds, worried out of his mind. Fortunately there was no blood, but I really had banged my head hard. Blood platelets don't stick together to clot the blood when you have chemo, so I spent the rest of the night worrying that I had an internal bleed. There was no way I was calling the ward as I knew they would want me straight in and I was too angry and upset to be able to deal with them.

I have found that when I am in a state like this I only want trusted people around me. I was furious that these things were being done to my body and I didn't seem to·have much say about it – the last thing I wanted was to be delivered back into the hands of the people perpetrating the discomfort. Fortunately I had a blood test booked for the next day and would hopefully be able to deal with the situation a little more calmly then. My nose wasn't streaming blood so I figured I was safe for a few more hours yet.

Wednesday dawned bright and sunny and Lyn came to collect me for my weekly bloodletting. I was very glad she was, as my heart was still ricocheting around my chest and my poor bruised head was hurting. I was still very low and together we discussed our strategy for the hospital. I was so pleased she was there to support me as I didn't feel strong enough to run the gauntlet of the medics on my own. I felt the issue was that the new heart drug I was on was not only not stopping my heart from going into an irregular heartbeat episode, it was doing something to my system which was creating the sickness and dizziness once it had – which had never been there before with such ferocity. The blood tests are usually followed by the appointment with Catherine, the MacMillan nurse, who does a fabulous job of co-ordinating a cancer patient's needs. I told her what had happened and asked that she find a doctor for me to talk to as a matter of urgency. She was brilliant. Within minutes she had one of my doctors from Ward 11 in the room and we started negotiations. We went round in circles for several minutes as he wanted to keep me on the higher dose of Bisoprolol. One of the side effects of this drug is dizziness and sickness. Amazing isn't it? What are they thinking when they create these things? I, quite naturally, wanted to take the lower dose. Or none at all.

He parried with, "I think we should give you another tablet which you take when the attack happens, as a one-off, and stay on the high dose of Bisoprolol."

I replied that I am happy to try this new one-off tablet if I can stop the other one or drop the dose. I do think I have some logic going here, and as I am the one getting the horrible side effects I am determined to carry on. A smile and wink from Lyn confirms this. We carry on like this, and eventually I conclude that we are saying the same thing – he wants me to take another drug because this one isn't working. EXCELLENT.

I learnt long ago that the basis of good negotiating is to start from a point of agreement. Moments after that he agreed to drop the dose, and said that he just had to speak to the cardiologist to confirm it was OK to try the new tablet.

Fast forward – back in the waiting room and the doctor returns from his own negotiations – I can't have the other drug yet because it might not be right for my particular problem, so I will need to have a 24 hour trace sometime next week. I point out that now would be a good time, if ever, as my heart is currently misbehaving in a spectacular fashion and it would be wonderful for them to work on a scan of that. Next week it would probably be very well behaved and we wouldn't get the same result.

Fast forward another few minutes and we're called in to see the next doctor down in the pecking order to collect the prescription for the lower dose drug and organise the heart trace. Bless him.

His opening gambit was "I don't understand why you feel the need to drop the dosage. We would like to keep you on the higher level."

Oh no. In my fragile state I had to go through it all again, only this time I was getting angry. I asked him how he could possibly expect me to have any kind of a life when apart from dealing with the effects of chemo, I also have to now contend with being totally incapacitated and needing 24 hour care for 2 days every week or so, because I am keeling over from the drugs that they insisted I take. Which weren't working anyway. Lyn moved in with a final thrust of support and he wrote the prescription.

Next stop ECG, where I was trussed up like a turkey with the heart monitor. The sensors had to be interwoven with my tunnel lines, then all the cabling hidden under my t-shirt, with the magic black box clipped to my waistband. Walking Frankensteina doesn't begin to describe it. Once free of the hospital, we thought we would take a jolly down Christchurch High Street just for a laugh to see if I could do so without tripping over my own cabling. I did, and Lyn bought me a lovely lunch.

I am sure you can imagine that all of this is very damaging and intrusive, even for someone who is well, but it isn't an experience that can be avoided or stopped, once it has started. You just have to deal with it. My big challenge seems to be in learning to deal with these events from a place of calm, or mindfulness, so that worries about the future and what may/may not happen, and whether or not I have control over it cease to affect the present moment.

With this in mind, and in great need of inner calm (heart still jumping about) I went joyfully the next day to see my friend Crispin for some sound therapy. If you haven't done this, try it. It is truly an experience sent straight from heaven. The first time I had a treatment I was reduced to tears by the sheer beauty of the sound. This isn't like a gong, or chanting, or anything you can possibly imagine. It is the music of the spheres incarnate. If in some greater realms there are lofty celestial halls thronged with wise, loving souls, then this is their backing music; no ersatz, horrible lift music for them, oh no. This glorious sound truly sings the soul back home.

I laid on the floor within a pattern of crystal and glass bowls, positioned so as to align with the chakras; other acoustic wooden and metal instruments are also used to enhance the process when appropriate. Struck firstly one by one (with a wooden stick covered in suede), the bowls are then eventually used in combination to produce stunning harmonies which last for an eternity. The sound goes straight through me, into my very bones. This time I also saw colours.

Careful readers from previous blogs will note that I am on a journey of introspection and I was interested to see what this healing session would produce. When Crispin got to my throat chakra I was expecting a very strong reaction as it is not only the site of the cancer but also the place where I feel most blocked. (Obviously). This means that anything emotional tries to come pouring out, which frankly can be a very unpleasant feeling as I want to both release and block at the same time. It is always a battle and I don't enjoy it at all. I have done a huge amount of releasing, and the fact that there still seems to be a bottomless pit of emotion indicates to me that whatever I'm doing isn't working. This time was different though, and it only elicited a few tears, in a very gentle, 'Oh yes', kind of fashion.

The very clear message I was getting was to open up. I had already started to feel this in previous sessions of EFT and meditation so it was good to have it confirmed in such a beautiful and gentle way.

Introspection is all well and good but you still have to have a sense of direction: I am enjoying the experience of quietly watching to see what comes up, and to see where following that whisper leads me. So I was laying bathed in sound, wondering why I was finding it hard to open up. I saw myself, almost from above, as being closed and scared. Closed down, although I had done so much work in the past on letting go. Why? How much more can I do? But letting go is different from opening up, isn't it? Letting go is a release, whereas opening up is an invitation to visit. And are we brave enough to see who will come visiting? Enter the fear.

Once we start talking about fear and get over the obvious ones, fear of dying, fear of losing your job, partner, health, etc., you start to look at how fear actually affects your daily life, and how it might have been a pattern since early childhood – possibly rooted in some almost imperceptible slight or incident many years ago. My mum used to tell me how I had regular nightmares as a tiny tot. This grew into a fear of newspapers blowing in the street (there seemed to be a lot where I lived, near the marshes in Essex), men (?!), and loud noises.

What on earth was going on in my impressionable and unformed mind that could possibly have upset me so much, so young? I wondered how I would be able to find out, then I realised that it doesn't actually matter. I realised that I try to understand the world using logic a lot of the time.

Although I am a Cancer Sun and empathise in a watery fashion all over the place, my way of understanding any crisis is where my very left-brain, logical Virgo Moon runs amok. I think I do this too much. It occurred to me that what I am dealing with is something that doesn't necessarily have an *answer. I don't necessarily need to know that a particular event, either in this life or a previous one, has created the reaction of fear in me, and it is that I need to spend time with. I have spent huge amounts of time going back to forgive, integrate, acknowledge events and people that have hurt me in the past, and in past lives. You name it, I've done it, and for me, that strategy (good Virgo word) isn't working. I am watching a beautiful presentation by Thich Nhat Hanh on mindfulness and fear. It is the worry about the future (which is pointless) and sadness or regret for the past (which we can't change) that intrudes on our present and I know I am guilty of both.*

Both Stephen and I are finding that our world is changing tiny bit by tiny bit, on a daily basis. We have always talked about these kind of things but our conversations now have a passion and vigour they didn't before. This isn't just armchair philosophising or intellectual discussion. This is a real life situation that needs more than just band aid and placations, and it offers, as nothing has before, a massive opportunity to explore our inner landscapes and wonder at the complexity and the potential contained within. As Joseph Campbell said, "We must be willing to get rid of the life we've planned so as to have the life that is waiting for us." Amen to that.
Happy Sunday,
Margaret xx

So much for introspection – I was rattling around happily in my head, unaware that my cell count was plummeting. The next blood test showed I was neutropenic, which means that my white blood cell count, i.e. my immune system, was zero, as a result of the chemo. I was wide open to any infection and all of a sudden had to take precautions akin to going on holiday in a very dirty country. Eat only fruit that could be peeled, no salads, no runny eggs, nothing reheated, no rice (harbours bacteria unless punishingly hot)... the list went on, and included a ban on going shopping or receiving guests as it would be very easy to pick up an infection from other people. The guest bit was particularly horrible; my sons only spend part of the week with us, and this meant they had to stay away. Although we kept in touch on the phone, I was desperate for some mother-son hugs. They had to wait. I put out an SOS on the next blog and received powerful and beautiful healing in return. So powerful that when I went back for another blood test, my cell count had soared.

Cell Count

Blog #15 19th February, 2013

This is more of an interim note that a full scale blog. Went to the hospital on Monday and apparently my white cell count has plummeted despite all the supplements and the GCSF injections. It was absolutely fine last week but the last cycle of chemo does have this effect. What this means is that I am wide open to infections so I am on house arrest until Thursday, when I have another blood test. If the white cell count is still low I will have to go in for blood platelets or a blood transfusion, neither of which I want.

Luckily I can work remotely from the desktop at home - but the crazy thing is that I really do feel fine. It was a real shock to be told how much my blood count had dropped and for a while I felt really angry with my body.

Which is a pointless exercise I am sure you will agree.

There does seem to be a message in all of this about insisting on continuing on as normal when my poor body is protesting that it needs a break. Maybe this time I'll learn! Our lovely flat is filled with sunshine, so I am planning on sitting in my own little spot of it and absorbing the light and goodness. No doubt that will manifest as another blog, but in the meantime, for those of you kind enough to be sending me healing, I would be truly grateful if you could focus on the regeneration of my white cells.
Thank you so much
Margaret xx

The fabulous thing about being brave enough to open up on the blog was that having done it, people were only too happy to send healing. It was impossible not to be lifted by messages like these.

Dolores:
Ok Margaret...one load of regenerated blood cells coming up, courtesy of the Archangels.

Mario:
Your white blood cells will regenerate as if by magic, Margaret. You won't even know it's happening!

The Only Way is Up!

Blog #16 21st February, 2013

Dearest everyone, thank you so much for all your chanting and healing energy. I went to have my blood test today and my white cell count has gone from 0.9 to 48. In 3 days. Yes. How absolutely totally incredible is that? Stephen (cynical Virgo – no!), did wonder whether they got the decimal point in the wrong place last week, but I'm happy either way! The doctor did say that levels can "really shoot up" with the GCSF injections but even she was surprised at quite how much mine had. She of course has no idea of the enormous amount of healing that has been coming my way, and I wouldn't expect her to even begin to understand it. She seems nice though, so maybe on the ward we will get around to having a bit more of a chat and I can test the water a bit. But the main thing is that it is well above 'excellent' and for that I thank you all from the bottom of my heart. I need my platelets to be a bit better populated too so if you have the odd moment that is the next point of focus, but I am on now track to start my next cycle of chemo next Thursday.

I had a totally mad piece of head-wear arrive in the post today from the lovely Judy (who has been commenting on the blog from her holiday in Egypt), that I opened and tried on when on a high from the hospital visit. I think it is for a bellydancing outfit, and I got Stephen to take a picture as evidence of just how happy I am at the blood test result.

I bumped into Dot on my way into the ward, and she was very sweetly telling me about the right kind of diet for neutropenia (which I'm not any more, yay!), which was very interesting. Given that people with low white blood cell count are supposed to have hot, well-cooked food it does somewhat question the wisdom of taking such people into hospital. Yes, it does protect them from the bugs and germs of the outside world, but how can hospital food possibly help them get better? Hmmm. I hear James Martin was involved with hospital food a while back, I wonder what came of that. I might email him to find out.

I must admit I have had a couple of days where I was on the verge of calling the ward to see whether I should go in. Having an itchy throat and headache is very bad news when you are neutropenic, but for me the prospect of the lack of sleep and horrendous food made it a lot more complicated. Stephen was very worried, but I promised that if things got too bad I would call them. I really, really wanted to stay home with a passion, and, thankfully, I managed to. I wanted to have home cooked, good quality food most of all, and sleep with no interruptions a very close second.

It made me think again about how important it is to feel nourished on many levels when we are ill, and how none of that is addressed in hospital. For instance, Dot's heart is in the right place, but I think that somehow the patients have been shoe-horned into the hospital schedule rather than the care being patient-led. That sounds like a really good, but unlikely, management phrase, doesn't it? It has just occurred to me that there are patient questionnaires all around the hospital so I think I might try to get hold of one of them and see exactly what they are asking about. I really, really doubt whether they ask, "Please score the quality of hospital food on a scale of 1 to 5…". I would so love that one. However, I will see whether there is any other way of giving feedback. I doubt I can do much about the food, but I was talking about the constant interruptions and early wake-ups with the nurse taking my blood this morning, and she said I should tell someone about it. Then she said she would too as it was really important. Her words were, "there is no way anyone can get better in hospital with all the early morning routines and interruptions".

Wow.

As I am in hospital next week I am going to try at least to see why they disturb us at such silly times and request whether some flexibility is possible. I think I already know the answer, but I am willing to bet that patients don't dare say anything so it has never seriously been considered before – I am willing to run the gauntlet! There is something so debilitating about being in hospital even if you are feeling well – I mentioned previously about changing into day clothes every morning so I don't feel so powerless, so I will wait for the appropriate moment when I am fully clad for the day. I might have my special pink belly dancing hat on just to disarm them :-).

The pink theme is really gaining momentum, and it really only started out as a bit of a joke with my two boys some time ago – I had to do something to counteract the massive amount of testosterone belting around the house, so I started very slowly with the odd item and now it has grown to this! Last time I was in I had towels, flannel, toilet bag, soap holder, slippers, duvet cover, pyjamas, all in black and pink or just pink, plus the lovely knitted hats, Fenella Flamingo (pics below)… and I have since gained a pink wineglass and now Judy's pink hat…

And the medics seem to love it. It also makes me feel stronger too. I always place Fenella (who came with that name and whom I have had for about a year now – she isn't just a hospital flamingo) behind me so that they have to look at her when they are talking to me – you can see from her picture that she is really stern and will take no prisoners. I like to think that with all the pink influence the doctors and nurses feel they are coming into my area – call me deluded but I think it helps. Just to see them crack into a smile, or try to stay focused on me when they are also looking at a pink fluffy flamingo is priceless.

I want to say that I think I am getting truly amazing care at the hospital, and in no way should my comments be seen as a criticism of the wonderful people who are working so hard to make me well. What I am hoping is that I can inject a little more fun and life into proceedings while I am there, as we all know how important it is to stay positive.

Talking of being positive, feelings can run very high in the waiting room. Stephen and I were talking to a lovely old couple (80 and 84) who were there for the husband's treatment, the last of very many sessions during which he has had several remissions and relapses and had survived to this point, smile intact. I did see them as being inspirational, and although they appeared to be reciting a whole list of treatments, they were actually being very positive. Another lady present didn't see it as such, maybe she wasn't listening with both ears. She was called to see the doctor, and before going out, turned towards us, and then the elderly couple, and asserted, "It isn't always like this. It doesn't always come back. I've been clear for seven months. Positive mental attitude, that is everything. It doesn't have to come back." Then she stomped out.

I was horrified. I don't think I would like to live with her version of a positive mental attitude. Granted our new-found friends were slightly intrusive and I was beginning to miss the book I was reading, but I was angry that they had been so attacked by a stranger when they had been through so much, and they were simply sharing their story with us. People change when they are given a diagnosis for a life threatening disease, and they cope *with it in different ways. This woman was obviously fighting it with every fibre of her being, but it did make me wonder, where is the love and lightness in her soul? And in terms of cancer, I'm sorry, but seven months isn't a long remission, especially when compared to what this gentleman had been through. How will she cope if it comes back? Her so-called 'positive mental attitude' had actually rocked four people, and not in a good way. My heart goes out to her.*

Be happy and well!

Margaret xx

The waiting room and Ward 10 were where everybody's coping strategies were on display, and for the most part they were cheerful places. Membership of the Cancer Club is exclusive, but there is a spirit of openness and possibly even a siege mentality. The nurses, in particular, have a fabulous sense of humour and never fail to take the mickey out of each other, and the patients who can cope with it, when the opportunity arises.

However, there were storm clouds on the horizon. What more? Yes, on several fronts. After our lovely day out in Christchurch just over a week previously, Lyn had developed a really bad headache. She had seen the doctor several times (sound familiar?) but nobody had a solution. It was only when she saw an enlightened locum that she was sent to hospital for an MRI scan. After that she was blue-lighted to Southampton where it was discovered she had a neural aneurism – bleeding on the brain – which could have been fatal. She was rushed into surgery where she was operated on for more than six hours; nobody knew whether she would regain her faculties – only time would tell. It was a huge shock to me and Stephen as Lyn and John have given us such unstinting love and support through all this. The thought of losing either of them was almost too much to contemplate.

I was also becoming increasingly disenchanted with my treatment plan. I had been doing a lot of research, and there is no middle ground with cancer and chemo – people are either for or against, and the evangelists of alternative treatments have nothing but bad to say about chemo. Which is very hard to read when you are the one going through it. It all unravelled in the next blog.

Changes Afoot

Blog #17 2nd March, 2013

You might have noticed there have been no posts from hospital or accounts of exciting encounters with Dot. After a recent blood test which showed just how healthy my bone marrow is, I had a kind of awakening. The objective of this particular chemo is to destroy almost every cell in my body (a few cancer cells, but generally also a lot of very good quality ones), then replace them with cells grown outside (stem cell transplant) with the hope that my body rebuilds itself.

I came out of the appointment wondering why on earth I was doing this. The quiet whisper has become a roar and I can no longer avoid it. The shock and speed of my diagnosis left me no time to explore other options, and, fearful and panicked as I was, I leapt almost whole-heartedly (but to be truthful, with a lot of apprehension) into the treatment regime that appears to be my only hope. I might be pink and bouncy when I am in hospital, but underneath all that I have extreme doubts about this treatment and especially the side effects.

We're not just talking hair loss and nausea. The possible side effects are included on the consent form I had to sign before treatment started, and the registrar apologised that he had run out of space but I could have a further booklet to enlighten me if I wanted to know more. Included in those that did fit on were heart failure, arrhythmia (like I need more?!), sudden death, liver failure, kidney failure, permanent brain damage, liver/lung changes – oh, and failure of treatment. So I could go through all that and still not be well. My instinct that this poison was, well, poisoning me, was absolutely spot on. I haven't looked at the statistics of the people suffering from side effects, but I have never been much of a gambler; if there is a chance I could get any one of those things I would rather not throw the chips down, thank you very much, so the whole scenario has been very much on my mind.

This whole episode was also heightened by several people mentioning the possible use of medicinal cannabis for the nausea I was complaining about. Of course cannabis is illegal just about everywhere in the world, and not because a very small percentage of people get off their heads on wacky baccy.

Oh no. Cannabis is illegal just about everywhere because it poses such a massive threat to several massive industries including Big Pharma. There are literally hundreds of case histories showing how cannabis oil has treated cancer, but you have to do a lot of illegal things to be able to use it, which isn't my particular strength. I get stopped going through Customs with just hand luggage, so I'm not about to get into anything even slightly illegal as they will come here first. Plus we have a policeman living just over the way, and nice as he is, I think he would probably want to investigate the source of the sweet smell emitting from our apartment. Go Google Rick Simpson if you are interested to know more.

This started to get me ever so slightly frustrated. The truth is I have such a rare and aggressive form of cancer that they don't have a neat régime for it like with other cancers. I know there are countless people alive today who are grateful for their treatment, but basically treating me is a work in progress which has lots of caveats and a fair amount of crossed fingers.

Thinking about the cannabis oil led me to other alternative therapies. My mum fought breast cancer for a second time with alternative therapy after an horrific encounter with radiotherapy when she first had the disease. That was 27 years ago and she survived longer than most women on conventional treatment at the time although, sadly like them, she did eventually succumb. In fact yesterday was the 20th anniversary of her death. Hi Mum! So I do know a bit about it, and it has definitely played a part in my health choices ever since.

A contact of Stephen's sent a lovely email wishing us both well and suggesting some herbs that might help me as well as details of a medical herbalist we could talk to. By this time my chemo appointment was drawing close and I was feeling more and more strongly that I needed some thinking space. At my pre-chemo appointment on Wednesday I said that I needed to delay the treatment until next week due to work commitments (partly true). There was no struggle but it was a hard thing for me to do as although inside I am quite a rebel, on the outside I am a real scaredy-cat. Anyway I managed it, and on Friday we were on our way to see an ayurvedic medical herbalist.

Apart from the glorious sunny weather, driving through one of the prettiest parts of England was a balm to my soul and we had a very useful appointment with her. She suggested an intensive 3 week treatment that would be taken in India called panchakarma shodhana. We're not talking

Indian Spa here – it is a seriously uncomfortable treatment that is designed to force the toxins from your system. I am still investigating the possibility of going to India, but I have already started on the slow version here. I left with my bag of disgusting tasting herbs and tinctures. I am following a 75% green veg no fruit diet (cancer cells love sugar), so basically any plateful must have 75% greens. So I am having really odd breakfasts like poached egg on steamed spinach and poached haddock on spinach and curly kale and I have just started fruit-free green shakes. I'll report back on that one! Curly kale of course being the latest big fad since spinach. Did you know that spinach isn't any better for you than any other greens? The scientist apparently got his decimal point in the wrong place and for decades we were duped into thinking spinach was especially excellent. See… never trust the science :-).

I haven't yet decided which route I am going to take. Astrologers amongst you will know that it is Mercury Retrograde at the moment. For the uninitiated that means it is a very bad time to make decisions. It is a time of research and investigation and of pondering. We have a meeting with the consultant on Tuesday in which I am going to suggest I take a 3-month break from chemo to investigate other methods of healing and discuss with him my very deep-seated concerns about the treatment. I will have Stephen there to help back up the scaredy-cat, don't-want-to-upset-people side of my nature. What does seem wrong though is that I should even worry about bucking the system. You could say, and no doubt many will, that I am considering refusing something that science proves works. The reality is that very big money funds the science with a vested interest to show that it works, which is absolutely not always the case. Anything ever so slightly threatening to these organisations has been stamped out by the 1939 Cancer Act. Read the inspiring but truly horrific case history that is going on as I write, to discover what we are up against http://sallyrobertsourstory.wordpress.com/sally-roberts-story/

I started this blog many posts back saying that I wasn't angry and that for me it was all about acceptance and surrender. I have found in the last week that I am actually becoming very angry; I am angry that I am being shoe-horned into a treatment that may not be in my best interests, and that options that may work better for me have been hounded out of town so they can't compete. I am also angry that I have to put a huge amount of effort into doing all this when all I really want to do is get on with life. To this

end I am becoming increasingly enamoured with Thich Nhat Hanh and the
way he teaches Mindfulness. I am reading his book Fear *because of course I*
am afraid. I face a very uncertain future and that is very scary. In Fear, *he*
teaches that we have to come back to the 'here and now' as this is the only
moment in which we can be fully present. The past has gone and tomorrow
isn't here yet, but I am here now. The poem I want to leave you with is one
that I have just started working with to help me understand and dispel this
anger. Anger and cancer are not good bedfellows. So we end up back at ac-
ceptance. Sometimes I astound even myself :-).

I have arrived, I am home.
In the here, in the now.
I am solid, I am free,
In the ultimate I dwell.

Be well,
Margaret xx
Chapter 9

The herbalist lived in the heart of the Cotswolds, an exceptionally beautiful part of England where little streams run along in front of picture-perfect cottages.

After the intensely medical, left-brained approach of convention-al medicine it was an absolute joy to sit in her office and talk about me-me-me for an hour. Ayurvedic medicine differs immensely from its allopathic counterpart in the west. Every comment, every feeling is noted, as well as tongue diagnosis and the taking of the pulses which ascertains how the energies are balanced and working (or not working) in the body. I have relied on herbalism and acupuncture on many occasions in the past when western medicine has failed to di-agnose or treat what ailed me. It has helped me with ME, tonsillitis, PMS, irregular heartbeat… Could this really cure my cancer? I had a lot riding on this.

The office looked out on an idyllic herby kind of landscape and the three of us were very much in the moment of a lovely spring day – and talking about me of course – when suddenly a pack of dogs ran across the garden, not 20 feet away; we all stopped in astonishment. The local hunt was apparently in transit and the hounds had followed the fox through the herb garden. There must have been at least 20 dogs, baying and crying. I was stunned. Where did all this fit into the scheme of things?

Being of a decidedly shamanic bent I believe that we can often be guided by animals if only we would stop and listen – but nothing had equipped me for this. In fact, it is only in looking back as I write this that I am considering the symbolism. My feeling is – with the wonder of hindsight of course – that the dogs did actually represent the chemo flooding through my system. However, at the time of the meeting I was filled with immense hope that the ayurvedic approach would work. I felt that a massive detox would balance the energies in my body and I could avoid any more damaging chemo. Of course the herbalist would not be drawn as to the possible success or otherwise of the treatment, but I left filled with excitement that I could go to India and be cured. On my terms.

We left the office and drove into Bourton-on-the-Water for our packed lunch; this village happened to be a great favourite with my mum, another bit of symbolism that was not lost on me. Here was I, sitting in one of the most beautiful places in the country, trying to decide on a course of treatment which would literally kill or cure me. To be honest, I was completely fired up, and ready to get the next flight to India, but in a way, thankfully, common sense did prevail. We munched our lunch in a thoughtful fashion, and I mentioned that I thought we should ask Komilla's opinion. Komilla Sutton is a very dear friend, and another lovely person that I can totally trust to talk sense to me when I would rather not hear it. As a vedic astrologer and a native of Northern India she would be in a very good position to help me make the right decision. She also has the incredible knack of always being at the end of the phone when I really, really need her (much like Swamiji).

Our picnic spot by the babbling brook was blessed with internet access (how weird is that, exactly?) so I sent her a message on Facebook. For someone of our generation that is also very weird, but I did it – needs must and all that. I had a message straight back from her. She was in transit through New Delhi airport and happened to see my message. She managed to call to my mobile from a payphone in the airport – how much more supportive can a friend be? – and after looking at my birth chart counselled patience and delay before making a decision. She was very concerned that I wouldn't cope with the change of culture and the strange treatment, which would be just as unpleasant as the chemo, only in a different way. She offered to call the doctor to talk it through with him, but was very insistent that I wait until at least the next Tuesday before making a decision. I reluctantly agreed and went on to the next call. If I was really planning on taking about six weeks off work I would need a lot of backup, and so called Cathy, who has been the office goddess in my absence. I asked if we could call in on the way home to discuss what we had learnt that day.

Her husband, Richard, is a superb negotiator and people person. After hearing the whole sorry tale he suggested that we have a chat with Joe to see what his take on it was. To say I was hostile to the idea would be putting it mildly as I knew from bitter experience that conventional medics usually hate anything that threatens their precious empire. I was all for just phoning in to say I was cancelling my appointment with him; however, as I just said, Richard has superb people skills, and by the time we left their house I had agreed to at least give Joe a chance to have his say. No idea at all how he managed that.

Even with a lot of help from Mindfulness practice, I was upset and frustrated. I wanted to get started on this! As soon as we got home I called Swamiji. We had a very fraught conversation in which she – surprisingly, from my point of view – encouraged me to continue with the chemo. I was gutted. How could my oldest friend and spiritual guide dare to side with Big Pharma? She had known my mum well, and pointed out that Mum would probably have survived for a lot longer had she combined her natural remedies with conventional treatment rather than completely rejecting it. That really hurt. I was full of enthusiasm for a system that could heal my body without the toxins, and I would hear nothing against it.

I called my brother, who uses alternative medicine wherever possible. I was sure he would back me up. He travels very widely for his job and he has a lot of experience in going to far-flung places that are way off the beaten track. Which this ayurvedic hospital is. He pointed out that I would need a whole load of vaccinations just to be able to get there – not a good idea in my condition – and in that condition, I would be finding my way from the airport into the mountains, then trying to adjust to an alien culture whose language I didn't speak, at the same time as undergoing some very unpleasant treatment. Quite apart from the fact that I would then return home (assuming everything went OK) to a situation where I was outside of any medical support system. This wasn't painting a pretty picture.

Fenella Rides Again

There was a very real danger, for a while, that Fenella might be retired to more of an observer kind of role. I was really, really, close to chucking in the chemo and going completely along the alternative route. This has been one rollercoaster of a week but I think progress has been made. As you know, I went to see an ayurvedic medical herbalist last week, and I have since been following a 75% green veg diet. Any meal I have, including breakfast, has to be 75% vegetables, the greener the better, and raw if possible. So I have been having a teeny bit of poached fish and a whole bag of organic spinach (steamed) for breakfast, and so it goes on through the day – and I have to say I feel really, really good. She also suggested a three week, seriously uncomfortable intense detox at an ayurvedic hospital in India. Even this sounded preferable to continuing chemo with all its attendant discomfort, but fortunately some very good friends prevailed and suggested a) delaying any decision for a few days and b) having a proper conversation with my consultant (which we hadn't yet had because it was all so rushed once I was diagnosed). So, much against my very cardinal instincts, we did both.

I phoned the hospital on Friday and managed to get squeezed in to see Joe on the following Tuesday. I have to say that when you have cancer people move mountains to help you, for which I am eternally grateful. With my incredibly sick sense of humour I wonder whether that is because they are never quite sure how urgent the matter is, but, whatever, I love it! So we pitched up nice and early for our meeting and I was really nervous. As far as I was concerned I was telling him that I definitely WAS having a break from chemo and going off exploring all these other wonderful ways of getting well, plus IF I ever needed to come back I wanted to be able to have one of these new treatments that is being tested and is apparently a lot less toxic. I was ready to wage war. Kind of sweet really, and very slightly innocent round the edges.

Joe was running over half an hour late and had more patients after us, judging by the waiting room, yet greeted us with a lovely smile. We were ushered to a really comfy room with sofas, and nice blinds on the windows, which is really quite unusual for the NHS, but very comforting, and then he gave us nearly an hour of his time – he would have sat there as long as we needed it. His phone was going crazy on silent vibrate in his pocket, but he completely ignored it. I was so impressed. I knew Joe was lovely anyway, but this was exceptional. He listened very attentively to all we said. He knows about all of the treatments I mentioned. He also knows a lot about ayurveda, being from Kerala, and was very supportive of it. His biggest worry is that Mantle Cell Lymphoma is so changeable and so aggressive that very few things kill it entirely, and it only takes one cell to remain for it all to kick off again. He was concerned that the ayruveda wouldn't get it all. After each treatment of chemo it morphs into another type of cancerous cell, which is why they have to cycle the chemo very aggressively in the beginning to reduce it bit by bit until it is all gone. Hopefully. Because of this I can't just take a break of a few months and go back to it – the cells will have adjusted to the treatment so far and will be resistant to it. I mentioned the other much less toxic drugs that are being trialled (which he also knew all about) and he said that they are still at stage 1 testing. They are being used on people who have relapsed and have no other choice; there is an outside chance they will survive, but there is a possibility they will either die from the cancer or from the drugs not working/being too strong, so he would not use them on me. He expects them to be on the market in about five years when their effects are better understood.

We discussed the toxicity and side effects. Joe can change the medication I get for the side effects if necessary and the nursing staff keep a very close eye on the toxicity – the serious side effects don't just appear in minutes so at the first sign of anything going wrong they stop the drugs and reassess the treatment plan. Thinking about it, they are always asking how I am feeling, so this must be why. However, the most important thing that came out of this part of the conversation is that Joe is more than happy for me to use ayurveda alongside the chemo to achieve the best results if I choose to continue the treatment. This was the major thing that annoyed me while I was in the ward – that nobody would even consider talking about supple-ments, vitamins, whatever. It was almost fingers crossed behind their back, which is what in a sense drove me to seek alternative treatment. He said if I choose to continue with chemo and give him a list of the herbs I am taking he will check that there are no problems with them, but he doesn't expect there to be any. Finally, I am listened to. Fabulous. I am so blessed to have him as my consultant. So I was left with a different question from last week, one that is a lot more brutal. Either I continue with chemo, with all the things I am worried about but backed up by ayurveda, homeopathy, oxygen therapy, sound healing, diet, etc., thereby having a lot of strong therapies on my side against the bad boys, or I just take the alternative route and rely on myself to find a way through this and burn my bridges with chemo. Bit of a no-brainer then. I had to face the stark reality that if I chose the alternative route I wouldn't have any one person (who didn't charge by the hour) on call and able to advise and treat me if necessary. I could come back from India and be ill for any number of reasons, and be completely alone. When you have a life-threatening illness that is not a good option.

Our chat with Joe seemed to me to be offering the best of both worlds. I can throw the entire arsenal of ayurveda AND chemo at the cancer cells and Ha! They shall die! So Fenella's contract is safe and all the pink stuff comes out again as I go back in for Cycle 3 on Monday, along with all my green food. Do you like the way I'm building up a colour scheme here? One of the really clever things Joe did was get inside my head. It is a really confusing place for me, so I don't fancy anyone else's chances, but he was right in there. The survival rate for this kind of cancer is now 60% at five years. It used to be slightly above zero. The reason it is only five years is because the drugs have only been used for that long (duh, thank you Judy for explaining that to me. I thought they were all dying at five years!). In reality, when the next report comes out they are expecting seven years, then ten years, then after that you are considered cured. I have to say that I am expecting to be in that 60% of course. He suggested that if I can put up with 6 months of pretty horrible treatment supported by whatever means I choose (less actually as I have already started) then at least I have the rest of my life to go off on detoxes, and he said he is expecting me to live to 80. You can't believe how good that feels. When you look at it that way it is a whole lot more positive. Sprawled by a pool in somewhere wonderfully exotic is a lot more likely after this than a detox, I have to say, but the idea is the same.

When I look at the tumult that was the last week I am relieved to be where I am now. The diagnosis was such a shock that I was launched into the chemo without having the space to think. For every moment I delayed I imagined more cancer cells powering through my body, then when the reality of the chemo hit home I rebelled against the toxicity and veered off in the opposite direction. I really needed to do this, and I am so grateful that I have Stephen and some very good friends to contain and support this totally nutty side of my personality. What has come out of it all is that I now feel I am making an informed decision about my treatment, and that I have a consultant who will allow me to embrace the best of both Eastern and Western medicine to beat the cancer. I feel more empowered than I could have imagined and can even feel positive about the chemo that will be coursing through my veins come Monday. I have decided to call it 'happy juice' instead of poison and toxins because in the end I will be happy and well, and I WILL be lying by that pool!

How exhausting. I really feel for all my friends who support me through this. There is going to be such a party in the summer…

Just to wring a bit more emotion out of it all, I have been reading more of Thich Naht Hanh's book Fear. *It is the kind of book to read just a few pages at a time because you want to go off and practise what he is teaching. I was talking to Stephen about the latest little segment and about how by being in the present moment there is no past and no future, and suddenly the floodgates opened. He is quite used to this with me so he just stayed really calm and asked what happened. I had suddenly realized, mid-sentence, that by living in the present I was freeing myself from the past, and the immense release of that brought on the tears. How many of us carry around the past as some massive rucksack, that most of the time we don't even realize we are humping around? Freed of the past, who are we?*

That's it for now… there will be more soon as I have to reconnect with Dot and explain why her fridge is full of my food, and I know you will want to hear about that. But for now, trust me, the future is very, very pink.
Be well
Margaret xx

Exhausting, to be sure. But as several people on the blog pointed out, I had a sense of control back, and that was incredibly important. There was also a general sigh of relief that I had decided to stay with the chemo. Something that was brought home to me with great force is that whilst I might disagree with a lot of the tenets of modern medicine, at least in the UK we are blessed with free treatment. If I had chosen to follow the ayurvedic route, or any other alternative therapy for that matter, it would have cost a huge amount of money that we don't have. You could say I was stuck between a rock and a hard place as I was choosing the treatment that is better provided for in the West rather than the one I felt most drawn to intuitively. But a decision had to be made. I realised that I did in fact feel safe continuing with the chemo; a strange sentiment maybe, considering the poison that would be pumped into my system, but it was good to know that I had a hotline to several people, at any time of the day, should I start to feel ill. And there were whole teams of people dedicated to looking after me when I went in for treatment. Consequently I was feeling much more cheerful and committed than in the last few weeks, and I was almost looking forward to getting on with the next cycle. If you can do such a thing. It didn't quite go according to plan though.

19. Halfway to Paradise

Blog #19 20th March, 2013

Apologies for the big delay in doing the new blog. I started writing this on Sunday, all full of the joys of incoming spring, whittering on about what a strange week it had been and how time is flying so fast that nobody can keep up with each other anymore... then on Monday my heart kicked off and I was completely out of action for two days, as was Stephen as he had to look after me again. Same thing as before – heart goes out of rhythm and I am not only completely unable to stand up without passing out but also incredibly sick if I do make it into an upright position. I had a hospital appointment for bloods etc. that day which we managed to delay until Tuesday, with the expectation that I would feel a bit better. So wrong.

I woke up the next day with all of Monday's problems and total weakness – I found it hard even to sit up enough to hold a drink as it was too heavy for my arms, so Stephen wisely got me to hospital. The nurse hooked me up to a saline drip and I used the bedside table to prop my arms and head on until the doctor came as they were just too heavy to carry. Whilst I was in that position – after about half an hour – I realised that my heart had gone back into rhythm, and by the time the doctor came back with my blood test results I was starting to feel almost perky, and I had stopped resembling a ghost. We all thought I might have been anaemic, but the battery of blood tests showed my platelets are fine (although I am neutropenic again, which is hopefully just a temporary glitch) so there was no obvious reason for the sudden debilitation except possibly dehydration. And my heart. I am happy to report that not only was I able to walk to the car to go home (having been brought in a wheelchair, much to my chagrin) but today I feel almost sprightly. So there we go. That was the short excuse for the delayed blog :-)

But I do have to catch you up on the last chemo session (last Monday/ Tuesday), which was memorable for several reasons, and I know you would hate to miss it. That bit of the week went v-e-r-y slowly. I started Cycle 3 (which is the same as Cycle 1) on Monday morning at 11.00 and finished several litres of liquid later at 3.30 the following morning. That, in my mind, is way too long, and I shall be having words when we get to Cycle

5. When I was finished with all the chemicals, the nurse left me on what is called a slow flush, a drip of saline solution which keeps the Hickman lines open. This means the staff don't have to go rummaging around in the wee small hours to make them all sterile again which is really quite a procedure. I am sure she meant well but come 6 o'clock I was still awake as I can't seem to sleep when I'm hooked up. Then, skip this bit if you have a weak stomach, I got up to use the bathroom and was violently sick, over and over again for what seemed like ages – so I couldn't even pull the bell for help.

When I finally stopped and took a moment to splash my face with cold water I was horrified by the vision that greeted my eyes. The undersides of my throat were huge, like a hamster storing all its winter provisions in one go (I guess that is technically cheeks, but just go with me here), and my eyes had massive swollen bags under them. It was quite a shock, I can tell you. I got back to bed and buzzed for the nurse, who told me I would have to wait for the doctor to come round at 9.00. I wasn't impressed, given what Joe had said the week before about keeping an eye on side effects. I did feel better for all the evacuation though and amazingly managed to get about an hour's sleep before the next interruption. I was absolutely, definitely planning on going home that day, so I spent a lot of time talking myself out of being ill; the last thing I wanted on ward rounds was for them to keep me in. As it turned out, an injection of anti-histamine took most of the swelling away and I managed to escape as planned.

So what does one think about in the endless hours on a drip? If you have been following the tortuous journey so far you will know there has been a shift in my attitude, and this was a good place to test it. This is the first treatment where I have felt fully involved and positive. My emotions previously were fear and absolute hostility, but armed with my ayurvedic remedies, the vast amount of healing being sent to me and my healing meditations on the iPod, I felt as if I was only now embracing all the options open to me to beat this cancer. And it felt good. Tiring, for all the reasons above, but a lot more positive than previously, as I visualised all the forces working together to get the chemo through my system and into every single cell that needed to be blasted into oblivion.

Even the violent sickness was good in a perverse kind of way as it was a very quick method of getting some of the toxins out, although I'd prefer not to do that again too soon. That was weird too, as once it had served its purpose it just stopped – job done. I was also aware that I am now halfway through the treatment. I'm not going straight into the stem cell transplant as I'm hoping it won't be necessary, and it can be done at a later date if it becomes so. When all this is over and the dust has had time to settle a bit, Stephen and I are booking ourselves into a 5-star spa resort we have seen on Santorini, for some much needed rest and recovery. Long days of sunshine, sleep and good food, with not a drip or hospital meal within miles. We can't wait!

Mercury's retrograde journey back through Pisces has been incredibly testing for everyone, but on a personal basis it has enhanced my voyage of discovery. My Moon is ruled by Mercury so its position has a lot of bearing both on my thought processes and on my ability to articulate my emotions.

A few days ago I checked to see where it was on the day of the first visit to the consultant, in December. I was amazed to see it went into Sagittarius on that exact day – which perfectly describes my path of spiritual self-examination, my need for answers from outside of myself, and my exploration of other disciplines from around the world that can help me.

During its time in Pisces I have been considering and agonising about toxins and side effects of the drugs, but Stephen and I have also been slowly overhauling both our diets and the products we are exposed to in daily life. We have especially been having a lot of discussion about water, because if I am supposed to drink loads of water to flush all this through my system I don't want to be taking in more toxins.

I'm completely aware of the tap water versus mineral water debate, but whichever route we choose I want to be quite sure our water doesn't contain everyone else's hormone/heart/statin medications, metals, pesticides, plus whatever else ends up in the system. I have quite enough problems without that. My mum did the whole water filter jug thing way back in the eighties, so I felt a bit of new research was needed to see what has been happening since. The answer is nothing. The same old jugs are still out there.

I happened to read a review of one on Amazon from a customer who said that despite her best efforts there were always carbon particles from the filter floating in the water. Yuk. Don't want those. Then it occurred to us – knowing that keeping water in plastic is BAD – that we were considering buying one of those dinky jugs that stores the filtered water IN PLASTIC in the fridge, with the filter hanging in the water. That was a real 'duh' moment.

Back to the drawing board. The upsetting thing about all this is that we are exposed to all these toxins in the course of trying to be healthy. Is it me or does life seem a bit hard work some days?

Anyway, our research showed that you either pay about £25.00 for a fancy plastic jug with a carbon filter, or you go the whole hog and install a five filter reverse osmosis system under the sink which guarantees to remove 95% of metals, toxins and other gunk from the water. This is more likely to cost about £250.00, so clearly a lot more thought and research needs to go into it from our end. We went back to basics and ordered a water quality tester on the basis that it is good to know what one is dealing with at the start. And I have just been having a play. There have been 'sensitive' moments in the past when we have offered bottled water to guests which has been turned down with comments like 'tap water's good enough for me' (I have never personally subscribed to this unless you know your tap water comes from the local mountains), so I was all agog to find out which is cleaner, bottled (in glass) or tap.

The purity of water is measured in the percentage of Total Dissolved Solids, which covers everything in water that shouldn't be there as well as a few bits that probably should, if it has filtered down through green and pleasant lands. The lower the TDS level, the more able your body is to be absorb and use the water and the few toxins it will have. The higher the TDS level the more likely the water is to be contaminated and thus be less beneficial to you. The acceptable maximum level is 500 Parts Per Million. Drum roll, results time: our tap water measured 239 PPM, which on http://www.tdsmeter. co.uk/abouttds.html registers as average tap water/marginally acceptable. Our Waitrose glass bottled water from organic lands measured 125 PPM, which qualifies as acceptable water from mountain springs. So I feel ever so slightly vindicated in buying the bottled version, but for the long term maybe we will invest in the under sink mega-water filter so we can cook with the water too.

Now I am feeling better I have a lot of other things to do before I go in for Cycle 4 after Easter, one of which is organising Hyperbaric Oxygen Therapy at one of the local MS centres. Oxygen given under pressure can help to kill cancer cells, which flourish in a low oxygen environment. It also helps the chemo work better, improves the immune system and aids healing. Chemo destroys all the good cells in your body as well as the bad, so I am up

for all the help I can get! The treatment involves taking a 'dive', sitting in a great big pressurised container, hooked up to a mask for about an hour, for as many times a week as I can manage it. Sounds brilliant to me – any excuse to sit for an hour and either read or meditate is incredibly attractive at the moment. The synchronicity from a previous blog comes to mind. I love the way the blogs have a life of their own and something I mention in one comes up later on in another. I'm thinking of Number 9. which was called 'Dive Deeply into the Miracle of Life'. I didn't know about HBO therapy then, so I love the symbolic link. While I am 'diving' I can also be meditating and generally pontificating on this truly mad, and hopefully miraculous metamorphosis I am undergoing.
Be well
Margaret xx

I can now say that at the time of writing we have sort of solved the water problem. We decided to invest in a High pH Natural Biomineral Alkaline water filter (about £50.00), which was producing lovely, sweet tasting water from our tap water, which is apparently better for us than either ordinary filtered tap water or bottled water. Given that cancer cells flourish in an acid environment we thought it would be a step in the right direction.

We were doing really well with it, then the rains came. December through to at least February saw gallons and gallons of water dropping from the skies; the flood plains did their job but the land was so saturated that nothing could drain away. Coincidentally, at the same time our water started to taste horrible – like it was stale and had been left out all night. We wondered whether the bad weather had something to do with it, so I called the water board and asked for someone to come out and check the quality of our supply.

The lovely guy that came out was really interesting and we learnt a lot about where our water comes from, which is in fact a local treatment plant. I was a bit disappointed about that. I know we don't have any local mountains to supply us with freshly running spring water, but I don't want to think about what goes in and what comes out the other end of a treatment plant. Somehow I don't completely trust the process. However, as it isn't practical to dig an artesian well in our back garden, we don't have much choice! The results came back to show that apparently our water is fine and has passed all the tests. It still tastes horrible though, so we're not quite sure where to go next. I guess we can't really tell what is going on until the water drains away and the surrounding area starts resembling countryside again.

When my heart wasn't playing up and I had recovered from the post chemo sickness, I was coping very well, and going in to work for a commendable amount of time. However, appointments at the hospital and investigations into other forms of treatment were swallowing up a lot of time as none of them were particularly straightforward – and it was taking ages to get going in the morning due to the vast arrays of supplements I was taking. Responses on the blog showed that folks wanted to know what I was taking, so I spent a lot of blog #20 on the exciting minutae of my daily preparations.

A Busy Old Time

Blog #20 29th March, 2013

I am still amazed how fast the days are passing, and how busy those days are. When we first started dealing with the chemotherapy I assumed that I would have days lounging around being incapacitated and bored, with enforced rest, but the reality is that there is always something to do – and I have to actually schedule rest time. Stephen laughs at that as he persuades me yet again to sit down and take it easy. Usually, unless I am really feeling bad, I am up again after about half an hour with my nose into something or another. Just getting sorted out for the day also takes quite a bit of time as I have a lot of things to take. There have been various enquiries into what I am actually taking so I thought I would share it with you.

First up is two tablespoons of Aloe Vera juice. We use the Pukka juice which is from the inner part of the leaf and is really soothing and delicious. Chemotherapy can cause permanent damage to the stomach lining so I am doing everything I can to protect it. In the interests of keeping my body in a more alkaline state we have either a slice of ginger in hot water for our first drink of the day or linseed tea with a slice of lemon. Have you tried that? It is lovely. It lubricates the digestive tract and calms down inflammation. It also makes it easier for waste products to travel through to their natural conclusion as it is kind of gloopy. Take a few tablespoons of organic golden linseed, add about 2 pints of boiling water, bring it back to the boil (watching it like a hawk as it boils over really easily and is impossible to clean up) then simmer gently for about 20 minutes. Leave it to cool down for an hour or so. Once it has done so strain it into a jug. The straining part is interesting as there is a certain element of it which stays so gloopy it is unstrainable and you have to throw it away. If someone out there can suggest a use for the bit you can't drink I am all ears, metaphorically speaking. We keep the jug of liquid in the fridge where it will be fine for up to 5 days. When you are ready to drink it put half a mugful in a saucepan to reheat then top up with boiling water and a slice of lemon. Delicious and very, very good for you.

After that and before breakfast I take two wheatgrass protein capsules, which support the immune system and a load of other things that have been shown to help destroy the cancer cells. It is available as a powder but I'm really not good with drinking pond water, which is what it does to anything you add it to. I also take 4 capsules of my ayurvedic powders which I had capsulised as they make even worse pond sludge. Chemo messes with your digestive system so much that I found I really couldn't tolerate drinking two glasses of the dissolved powders on an empty stomach. Breakfast is usually something like steamed spinach with a very small bit of steamed fish or a poached egg or two. The diet I am following is 80% vegetables and as much of that as possible should be dark green. Either spinach or curly kale, which is supposed to be the new spinach. Let's hope they got their sums right this time :-). Very occasionally I have porridge made with water and stir in a big tablespoon full of whey protein isolate. This is very good when my stomach is sensitive and I need more protein – it is easy to lose weight when you are on chemo.

After breakfast I take two capsules of turmeric (cancer fighting), a spoonful of my ayurvedic liquid, a capsule of Olive Leaf Extract (brilliant antioxidant and it helps to keep my heart and blood pressure under control) two Echinacea tablets, two teaspoons of Omega organic oil (flaxseed etc. combo) into which I put one drop of Vitamin A and two drops of Vitamin D3. These drops, I am sure, are the reason that firstly I don't suffer with the mouth problems that chemo patients usually do, and secondly that my blood count recovers quickly after treatment. After that I take the boring hospital stuff, a few tablets of this and that.

Lunchtime is a lot less intensive with just the ayurvedic stuff before and after, and the evening meal the same but with more Echinacea and Olive Leaf Extract, followed by the oil but only the vitamin D3.

And it's not just the tablets that take time. Last week I had to go to hospital every day to have a huge antibiotic injection into my lines, because there was an infection brewing where the Hickman lines come out. That would be a very bad thing and could be why I was feeling very ill in the early part of last week. I generally try to stay away from antibiotics, but an infection can turn from annoying to life-threatening very quickly when you are on chemo with a compromised immune system, and I'm not silly enough to mess around waiting to see which way it would go. I opted for going into the hospital every day for a week instead of taking 4 doses of 400mg a day in tablet form as it would have completely wrecked my stomach. Anyway, as *a cancer patient you get free parking and a nice cup of tea or coffee (joking) and even sandwiches if you time it right (also joking). Dot has been mysteriously absent every time I have been in. No doubt I will get the chance to catch up on gossip at some point. And the infection has gone :-)*

I thought life would slow down a bit now the antibiotics are over but I found that won't be the case when I finally managed to get to the MS Centre to sort out the Hyperbaric Oxygen Therapy. I was incredibly disappointed not to be able to have a go, but this visit was to fill out forms; I'm now a member of the MS Society so will no doubt get a magazine every so often. If anyone wants it do let me know! It was also to let me see the 'diving bell' and discuss which depth I wanted to go to. The process is good for cancer sufferers as oxygen taken into the body under pressure kills cancer cells. I need to go as often as I possibly can to literally keep up the pressure. The centre is about a 40 minute drive from home, the dive lasts about an hour, then I will drive to the office, about another 40 minutes. As the dives are at 11.00, I should be in the office for about lunchtime on Mondays, Tuesdays and Wednesdays (assuming I'm not in hospital having chemo or sick at home), and I still have to schedule a rest. Crikey. Next week is especially busy as on Wednesday I have the HBO Therapy in the morning and blood tests and a meeting with my consultant in the afternoon. And a rest! Out of breath yet? I am... Anyway I digress.

The staff at the centre are totally nuts. Maybe they nip in and have a quick session when no-one is looking. The diving bell is also nuts. It is metal, big and white with seahorses and shells painted all over it. There are little windows through which you can see five people hooked up to two tubes each, doing every day stuff like knitting and suduko as if it was a perfectly normal activity for a Monday morning. You can't help laughing at the incongruity of it all. There are three choices of depth: 15 metres, 24 metres and 33 metres. I figured that as I have been thrown in at the deep end with this disease I might as well plumb the Plutonic depths straight away. Why paddle around in the shallows when you can dive straight in? Actually for my very first session I'm doing the 24 metres but then I'm booked into the deep one. And sitting in a metal container with other people doing their knitting and crosswords or whatever. Oh and the noise. Imagine five different rhythms of Darth Vadar breathing. I know I am going to absolutely crack up and I have no idea what happens when you laugh with pressurised oxygen going into your mouth and nose. Guess I am going to find out and I will of course share every detail.

So being ill is incredibly time consuming. My weekly schedule has suddenly been taken over by HBO, which combined with the weekly hospital appointment and the three weekly chemo sessions doesn't allow any time for me to feel unwell. Oh and when I first come out the District Nurse comes for eight days to give me a GCSF injection to boost my cell count, which I will have to co-ordinate with the HBO sessions. I would quite like to also fit in some more sound healing sessions and other types of healing but I have no idea when. I need a PA!

I hope any Wessex Astrologer customers reading this will understand how my time in the office is limited. I am so grateful to have work as a diversion and also as a lifeline. The very wonderful Cathy who is our book keeper and usually sticks to the numbers department of the business is doing an amazing job of moving over to the words department to help keep orders going out and correspondence flowing. I know she doesn't find it easy, just as I can't add up a column of figures and get the same answer twice. We work really well together because of our different skills and I am absolutely indebted to her willingness to step into the breach.

I often work remotely on the days when I'm not up to going in and this at least allows me to keep up to date and in touch with the most urgent matters. When I do go in it is all with the best intentions to leave early and have a rest, but it just doesn't work that way. I think having your own business is a blessing and a curse. I am focusing very much on the blessing part as it is wonderful to want to go into work. I can't imagine having a grindingly boring job as well as dealing with being ill.

"Why all the resting?" you might ask. I have been having daily blood tests to check the progress, if any, of the infection and last weekend the nurse said the tests showed that I was anaemic and would need a blood transfusion. For many reasons that I am sure you all understand, I absolutely, definitely do not want anyone else's blood unless it is unavoidable. We went straight to Sainsburys to buy liver and even more spinach. I am also taking Ferrous Phosphate tissue salts to help with this, but around the time of discovering I was anaemic I realised I hadn't taken any for a while. I am sure the two events are not unrelated, so I am religiously taking them now. I am happy to say that a few days later my favourite doctor mentioned that

I was a 'tiny, tiny' bit anaemic, but on looking at my notes we both realised that the platelet count had come up in the past few days, so whatever I am doing is working. He mentioned the 'T' word again and I said that I'd like to handle it with diet if at all possible, which was fine by him. I'm not saying that I have solved the problem as I'm not over it yet, but I don't understand why the medics rush to do a serious thing like a blood transfusion when a change in diet can probably achieve the same thing. So I am having as much liver and spinach/kale/broccoli as I can force down my throat. Fortunately I do like it, but 4 days on the trot (haha) can make Margaret a dull person, desperate for a change. The anaemia is the reason I have to rest. When I am anaemic I suddenly get really heavy arms and have to sit down, which is how I know I have overdone it. What me? Overdo things? Possibly, it seems. And it has to be a proper sit down with my feet up – sitting at a desk or doing a jigsaw puzzle doesn't achieve the same thing, probably for some complicated scientific reason. Thank heavens for books and my laptop.

Nearly forgot to tell you the most exciting bit, which proves to me that we are in the second half, where I hope, like in a football game, we get lots of 'goals' and score lots of direct hits on the cancer cells. Apparently Joe is really pleased with the way my system is recovering after every cycle (and seeing some of the poor souls in the waiting room, so am I) so he wants to harvest my stem cells after the next cycle in preparation for a possible stem cell transplant in the future. He has delayed that cycle (which should have been on Tuesday) for a week to allow me to fully recover from the antibiotics, which is lovely. I have this week to race all over the county to breathe lots of oxygen and eat lots of liver to get my platelets up. As I often observe to Stephen, we really know how to live. A week after Cycle 4 I go back in for another one day of chemo, then the day after that they hook me up to the machine that separates out the stem cells from my blood. The cells are then taken to Southampton by a motorbike courier with a flashing light (not really) to be frozen. This is real Frankenstein stuff.

For the harvesting procedure I will have to lay almost immobile on the bed for 6 hours while my blood is taken out of one arm, pumped through the machine then pumped back into the other arm. I do hope they get the flow rate right! Me and immobile don't usually appear in the same sentence and I'm not very happy about being unable to move my arms. You know that's when the itches will start… There is an option to have a minor procedure *to insert the necessary hardware into my groin, and although I rejected it initially it would be a lot better than not being able to move either arm. That would be like a vision of Hell, where there is food (and a book!) in front of you but you can't bend your arms to get it to your mouth (or eyes). Isn't it all exciting? All of this means that the next cycle – 5 – (SO close to the end!) won't happen until early May. This is fabulous news as we're are hoping to meet some very dear friends in Glastonbury at the end of April for some much needed R&R.*

Having this treatment means that I never know how I will be feeling from one day to the next so we can't actually book a hotel as we might have to cancel at the last minute – we will have to take pot luck on the day and hope that somewhere has a place, but just like everything else that is happening now, I am sure something will turn up.

That's it for now. I have loads more to write about but I will save it for the next blog – I'm off to put my feet up (as if...)
Wishing you a peaceful and joyous Easter,
Margaret xx

As well as belting off around the countryside in pursuit of oxygen therapy, I was also endeavouring to stay a tiny bit fit. Sue Joiner, a regular contributor to the blog comments page, had told me that a friend of a friend, also called Margaret, had also had Mantle Cell Lymphoma, and she was still doing well after seven years – a fact that she attributed to regular walking.

So walking shoes were dragged out, and as often as I could manage it, we strolled to our local beach. It also helped to bring back a bit of normality into a life that had turned very weird. Very often I couldn't go very far; chemo gets you like that. You think you are fine, then all of a sudden you need a major sit down in a very inconvenient place.

With a bit of imagination and careful planning we made sure that our walks had regular stopping places so I could recover for a few minutes. Some days were a lot harder than others, but something about the discipline of actually getting out there and doing something, even a tiny walk, helped to keep my spirit strong. As far as I was concerned, I wasn't ill, just temporarily and inconveniently incapacitated.

21. Diving a Bit Deeper

Blog #21 7th April, 2013

And so a period of relative freedom draws to a close. Tomorrow I go in firstly for an echocardiogram to check my heart is still looking OK, then upstairs to my good friends in Ward 11 to start Cycle 4. This is the same as Cycle 2 – 1 day of Rituximab, which takes about 4 hours followed by 2 days of Citarabine, which according to my blog #13 was pretty bad. It is great writing this stuff, but reading it back is a Bad Idea! One change is that I should be able to go home overnight after the first day as the actual drip doesn't last as long as the other 2 days, which are each 9am to 12pm then 9pm to 12am, when of course I can't go home. We are doing some strategic planning in the food department so I can have as little contact with hospital food as possible. According to my last blog I think I only had minimal contact with food anyway on the final day and that reappeared pretty quickly – so we probably won't waste our nice food on a two-way street if that is the case!

It is 4 weeks since the last cycle and a lot has happened in my head and heart since then. The mindfulness exercises have been hugely beneficial and I feel far calmer than I did – the wonderful thing being that you can do them anywhere and nobody will notice. For anyone that hasn't come across this, here's what you do. As you breathe in, a nice slow breath, you say to yourself 'As I breathe in I know that I am breathing in', then as you breathe out 'As I breathe out I know that I am breathing out'. Doing this in the middle of a frantically busy day or a difficult procedure really does give you a moment to reconfigure and get your bearings. I have come to see that some part of me loves being swept away into BusyBusyBusy mode which then becomes a self-fulfilling prophecy. I feel stressed and busy and perceive every interruption to be ramping up the pressure even more. I know I always was like this and no doubt got used to feeding off the adrenaline rush, but the difference now is that my throat starts to ache and I get very tired if I don't break into it periodically with a mindfulness moment. It is hard to believe that such a simple technique can make a difference but it does. There was a period a few years back where I used to come back from work and wrap myself in my meditation shawl and really seriously meditate for at least an hour. This happened to be a time when I didn't have anyone else around so I could take that luxury, but it is more difficult now. I find the mindfulness moments are more than adequate, and in some ways more beneficial. Having a nice long sentence for each breath does make you slow down and as Thich Naht Hanh points out, actually enjoy breathing. I am in a much better state to carry on working for a while once I have done this.

Something else I have been practising is focusing on whether or not I am available for someone to talk to or for a particular activity. Like so many of us, I'm sure, I have become very adept at multi-tasking. Not only is it very tiring – which I don't have the capacity for now – but it also means I'm not really paying attention to any of the things I am doing, or the people who are hoping for a sensible conversation with me. It is a concept discussed in Rachel Neumann's lovely book, Not Quite Nirvana and it is a technique taught to her children when they were at school. Brilliantly clever and I would love to have had the chance to use it with my boys when they were small. Rachel's children used to tap her on the leg, or wherever they could reach, and ask if she was available. This had the effect of making her question whether she could pay them attention or not at that particular moment. If she could, it meant stopping whatever she was doing and listening to them rather than only giving them half her attention, which children immediately spot and of course play up to.

The whole concept is interesting though because it does make you question what you are doing with that moment of time. Not the one you had a few minutes ago or the ones that are still to come. This one. And if you are fully in this moment there isn't space to worry about what is coming next. I have found this especially useful when I am thinking about forthcoming treatment – it is a double-edged sword to have been through the chemo cycle once. I have decided that knowing what is coming is very slightly worse than not knowing, and that effect is at least tripled when I have written about it and read it back by chance!

You could also interpret multi-tasking as a way of people-pleasing for those of us with wobbly boundaries. You don't say "No" to someone, you just expand a bit to include them or whatever it is they wanted. I learnt a bit more about this as you will see. I have been fortunate to have some fabulous healing this week: sound healing with Crispin, which took me completely out of myself and gave me a wonderful release from my physical body, and crystal healing with Jeni, which certainly gave me some revelations.

I need to digress a bit here. I woke up early the other morning and was fortunate enough to hear the dawn chorus. We have changed rooms recently to the back of the flat so the most we hear are the screaming seagulls, and my, are they screaming at that time in the morning! On this particular morning though, I heard a really sweet song. No idea what it was, sorry – really rubbish at identifying birds and their songs. I listened hard to the bird and moved into a spontaneous and totally relaxing visualisation. I'm not any good at the ones that are supposed to lead you into a meditation. I've lost interest by the time you have walked down the path, smelt the grass, appreciated the blue sky and found a place to lie down by a babbling brook... noooooooooo. This one took me straight into lounging in a gently swinging hammock in dappled shade. The temperature was just how I like it, the near-by sea a wonderful shade of blue, the bird was still singing, and everything in my world was perfect. I was also basking in the wonderful flow of healing that has been sent my way. How clever is my subconscious?

OK – so stay in the hammock if you will. No hardship there. I was having the crystal healing session with Jeni when I was asked to relax further and take myself to this lovely hammock by the sea, which I had mentioned to her earlier. As soon as I tried to relax, as opposed to it happening naturally as it had before, all the feelings of guilt, and 'I should be doing something not slummocking here' came flooding in as did a few tears at the realisation I was spending some time on ME. What became obvious is that I felt bad giving myself time out – not being available – and Jeni pointed out that becoming emotionally involved in that situation was counter-productive.

She asked me to step back so I could observe the emotion of the situation but said that I didn't have to feel it. I didn't need to actually be upset, which was a real change from other healings where I was allowing things to come up so I could 'deal' with them. After years of doing this I was quite frankly tired of getting so upset. It is also really physically exhausting and I need all my energy to get well. I realised that this reaction was following old habits and that if I was truly in the moment I could separate it from all those other moments where I had been upset.

Sounds easy but it was really hard, and I need to practise it so it flows easily, without effort. I get emotional very easily, whether it is picking up other peoples' emotions or my own spilling out when I would prefer them not to, so this technique will be a welcome relief from the habitual 'opening the floodgates' routine. I can also use it to distance myself from stressful situations that I would prefer not to deal with but have to – it is a good exercise in strengthening my boundaries and thus in looking after myself. In true Libra Ascendant style I have usually compromised in the past so that everyone is happy. I have avoided conflict at all costs as it makes me feel so bad, with the result that everyone except me gets what they want or need. Hmm. I wonder where that fits in with my illness? It isn't easy to change but the realisation that old patterns contributed to where I am now is a huge motivator.

As a further quest to better survive the toxicity of Cycle 4, I have just been using EFT to tell my subconscious that although the chemo is considered by some to be toxic, I trust it to target any remaining cancer cells and for it to leave my system safely with no side effects. The double-edged sword of knowing what to expect has served me well when I consider that it has helped me to gather some phenomenally powerful techniques. The irony of the situation is that I had to go through those first few cycles to find out what I needed to help me through the later ones. Talking of irony, I did have a laugh when I was with Jeni: before I arrived she had picked a card for me at random from a crystal oracle pack. The card? 'Joy and gratitude'. I had to laugh. She was obviously concerned at how on earth, in my current situation, she could possibly sell me this one in a positive light. We both had a good laugh, actually. But honestly, I can say that this whole experience is giving me a lot to be grateful for and joyful about. And I don't mean in a "Oh, it's a lovely day and the sky is blue" count your blessings kind of way (which irritates the hell out of me). I am incredibly grateful to the lovely people who have reached out with love and healing to support me and Stephen and our families, through all this. I am grateful that this experience has given me a new level at which to talk to people. It is like when a loved one dies, nobody knows what to say to you – but I am finding that as I break the ice with them about my cancer, they too experience a big release and are able to gain some healing from the situation. Almost everyone knows someone who had or has cancer, and they all have their stories, regardless of whether those loved ones lived or died. What this has given me is a greater reason and a more meaningful vocabulary with which to talk about the far deeper aspects of life, the ones that matter to me a great deal, than I had before. The joy I get from this is immeasurable, and I feel as though I am finally starting to find out what it means to be me.

A good example of this is the two sessions of HBO therapy I managed to get to this week. Picture the totally ludicrous situation where five ordinary seeming people pitch up at a therapy centre in the middle of nowhere. Instead of taking outer clothes off, everyone adds a layer. Outdoor shoes are exchanged for, on the whole, pink (yes!) fluffy slippers (except for the guy, who has fluffy walking socks) and when everyone is ready we congregate in the metal diving bell.

The door is closed and we sit around chatting as our ears pop, the temperature drops significantly and we 'dive' to 33 metres. Obviously we're not really going anywhere, for anyone who has just joined the story. At the mark "Masks On" we dutifully don our oxygen masks so obviously all conversation stops. Mostly. Two of my neighbours needed to discuss a particularly stunning chocolate cake recipe they saw in a magazine (difficult in a mask) but apart from that it is quiet for an hour except for the regular Darth Vader breathing of the assembled party. When the hour is up we take our masks off and chat for the next 10 minutes as we come back up to normal pressure. The difference is that although there was a certain amount of discussion around chocolate cakes there was also a lot of talk about what we are all dealing with.

These people were MS sufferers and the guy had permanent nerve damage due to a stroke and diabetes. Rather than turn into a pity party, what this kind of gathering does is allow you all to tell it like it is. Nobody is shocked, everyone is open, because we have all been dealing with our own dark nights of the soul, and it is so good to share it. Maybe the excess oxygen has something to do with it, but it was liberating to be able to talk to them, and a privilege to listen to their stories. Being seriously ill allows me to jump in at the deep end, because that is what everyone wants to talk about and what they are most scared of.

I've decided to leave the HBO therapy until after I finish chemo. The best results are obtained through regular dives, 20 sessions as close as you can have them. Trying to fit them between chemo cycles is likely to lessen their effect considerably so I will return in a couple of months. I will miss my new friends and the depths of our sharing as we dive... but I look forward to seeing them again as soon as I can.

See you on the other side of Cycle 4!

Be well

Margaret xx

The hammock turned out to be a powerful escape mechanism for me – maybe because the image was so strong and because it happened spontaneously. I love the sun, the sea, warm air, the sound of the waves as they hit the beach. Wrapping up for a breezy walk on the beach is one thing, lying in a hammock surrounded by gentle healing energy is quite another, and far more my thing. I had commented on this to Judy, who wrote back:

I'm filling in some of the blanks in the account I'm writing of our Egypt trip so I can put it on my website, the 'whys' that I haven't been able to look at before. So I'm revisiting Alan Richardson's Inner Guide *to Egypt. This really caught my eye in the light of what we were talking about yesterday, that calm space within:*

> *There is a magical technique – in all systems of Magic since the world was formed – in which a person can, no matter what his circumstances, create a 'secret place' within his mind. It can be a temple for specific meditative work, a place of escapist fantasy; or a simple quiet and utterly secure place within the mind where the individual can achieve a special kind of sanctuary. The magical temple [is] always something of a World Axis around which time, space and events are wont to spin.*

I reckon your hammock qualifies!

It is quite extraordinary, in a disconnected way, to read back through my experiences as they feel like they were happening to someone else. I know, from with Judy, that there was a lot going on in the background that didn't make it into the blogs – like our discussion of the hammock, which had much wider implications than I realised. She sent me a picture taken in Egypt of the Henu boat (which very strongly resembled my hammock), and followed it up with this, to be included in her article for *Kindred Spirit* magazine:

> *The shamanic journey starts with boarding the Henu boat, the great winged ship of Sokar (Osiris) 'the Lord of the Mysterious Realms' which floats not upon water but air and is powered by sunlight. So eager is it to fly that it has to be chained down when at a standstill. In*

The Inner Guide to Egypt, authors Alan Richardson and Bill J pose the question: "a sarcophagus is carried on board containing what?" and answer: "Ourselves."

The imagery was perfect. All the elements were there: water, sun and air. My spirit was yearning to soar with the eagles (always a favourite theme with me) but my body had to go through a personal kind of hell to be able to join it. There was to be no ducking out… I had to get through this treatment and be effectively re-born through the stem cell transplant. I loved this surreal dimension to my treatment and my personal growth, but you can understand it wasn't one that could be easily written about. Judy is passionate and extremely knowledgeable about Egypt and she resonates very closely with the myths, and the gods and goddesses. Her intention was to take the picture of me and Stephen to all the temples she visited and enlist the help of the resident deity to send me some very strong healing.

We had managed to stay in touch – somewhat sporadically – while she was away, but once she was writing up her experiences a couple of months later we were able to see how closely her dreams and visions were linked with my more earthly experiences. Cycle 4 turned out to be especially gruelling, as you will see further on, but there was one particular night when I had the most amazing dream, after which I felt refreshed and more able to cope. When Judy came to check her notes for that time, this is what she had recorded for that period. Sobek is a Nile god depicted as a crocodile, renowned for his protectiveness and healing, Hathor is the goddess of joy and femininity:

Eventually I moved, at Sobek's insistence, to a granite stela in a case behind him. Two crocodiles this time. Basking in the sun. Heads laid on rocks and tails hanging down behind. Sleepy. Chilling out. One eye on us (Terrie was with me) but unimpressed by these visitors from the 21st century. Hathor, depicted beneath them, was more welcoming. She and her priestesses gathered around Margaret, Terrie and myself in quiet communion offering their support and heart-felt wisdom. Margaret was in safe hands. So calm and restorative. A sisterhood. That's the way it has always been in my enduring friendship with Margaret, who has encouraged me to go deeper in my writing and, in turn, her wisdom has sustained me. We didn't even have to pay baksheesh to take photos, a rare event indeed.

121

I was especially low during this cycle as my body was becoming less able to cope with the onslaught of drugs. In the middle of the night I emailed her, and she came back with this. Talk about food for the soul. Self-belief has never been one of my strong points!

You are one of the most extraordinary people I know.
You are on an extraordinary and enlightening journey not just for you but for all of us who love you.
So be the best most extraordinary you today.
Be all those goddesses.
Be YOU

Cue tears… I was really finding out how if you open up to people they will support you. A big lesson for me, especially as I faced the certain discomforts of Cycle 4.

Are We Nearly There Yet?

Blog #22 18th April, 2013

Now I'm safely on the other side of Cycle 4 I can look back at the highs and the lows with a bit of perspective. You might be wondering how there can possibly be any 'highs' to chemotherapy. I would previously have questioned the sanity of anyone claiming such, but I am amazed on a daily basis at the revelations that come my way. The first bit of good news is that I had Day 1, the Rituximab, which only takes about an hour and a half, as a day patient on Ward 10, so was able to go home straight afterwards. Result! I went back in for Days 2 and 3 suitably equipped with Fenella, food supplies and duvet, feeling slightly higher in spirits at the prospect of only two nights in hospital.

As an inveterate people-watcher, you can imagine how this experience is giving me SO much food for thought. For the first time I was in the four-bedded ward right opposite the nursing station, and although I was moved later in the day and thus didn't have to experience the snuffles and moans of night-time, I loved it. In this cycle I am on the drip from 9am-12pm then 9pm-12am for two days, so have nine hours in between to kick my heels and generally wander around making a nuisance of myself.

On this occasion, on Day 2, I went down to the 'coffee' bar (I use that term more of a description of the place rather than the quality of beverage served of course) and sat reading my paper and trying to drink the coffee. Close friends know that Stephen and I like our cafetière coffee. We don't have a lot, but by heavens, what we do have is stunning, and to be honest nothing in any of the coffee shops begins to compare. So having a cup of coffee outside is more of a little thing to do to either rest from the rigours of shopping or, in this case, get off the ward. Needless to say, the coffee wasn't good enough to linger over, and having read my paper then exhausted the magazine shelves of the in-house W.H. Smith I soon found myself back on Ward 11. The three other ladies in my ward were in quite a bad way and needed a lot of nursing care. My previous incarcerations have always been in twin-bedded or single rooms, so this is the first time I have seen hands-on nursing on a grand scale, and here it was at its best. The NHS comes under a lot of fire in some areas, but, as I have pointed out before, the standard of care on Ward 11 is unbelievable. In the case of these three ladies the attention they needed was akin to a care home: in the space of a couple of hours the nurses had given two of them a bed bath, and the remaining lady a shower, hairwash, blowdry and a touch of makeup so she looked pretty for her husband's visit. I was touched to my core at the simple yet meaningful attention which had nothing to do with the training and technical ability of these highly trained nurses. The most seriously ill lady, Flo, was having severe breathing problems; she was put on oxygen and moved to a quieter area with all the love and respect you would wish for your nearest and dearest. I fear she is not long for this world.

You can imagine all of this made me feel even more of a fraud and a misfit. Where on earth do I fit into this world of sick people? When they moved me to Iso 2 to make room for all the male patients to move to the four-bedded bay I joyfully helped push my bed and accompanying paraphernalia along the corridor – a fact which didn't escape the attention of the nurses.

Cycle 2 (and thus Cycle 4) is like this though; the short dose of Rituximab doesn't seem to affect me much, and neither does the first three hour dose of Cytarabine. I think this is because after the morning dose I can wander around and the toxins work their way naturally out of my system. Alas it is a very different story after the night-time dose, which I have concluded just hangs around overnight, then at 8 in the morning I am being prepped for the next one so it feels a lot more like six hours straight. That is when I start to feel toxic and bad, and the bounciness of the previous day starts to become a distant memory. I nominated this as a 'duvet day' because I literally couldn't face moving. The nine hour gap between morning and evening treatments on this day has a completely different feeling, and I start to feel like Jekyll and Hyde. Yesterday I was all happy and bouncy and found time to talk to the other patients who couldn't believe I am actually ill. I think they thought I was some undercover agent with a different mission from their own. But make no mistake, on Day 3 all was not well, and I know there will be comments about this, but in a way I hate myself for this change.

Why can't I summon the resources to chase this stuff through my system in a timely fashion so I feel better? I don't know. I am surrounded by tools that will help; I have good food in the fridge (with Dot's blessing!), motivational and meditative music on my iPod, amazing books to read and I can't rouse myself to do any of it. It feels horrible. I spend the entire nine hours alternately dozing and feeling like I want to die, and the worse thing is I know I have another dose to face later the same day.

I have to confess I spent most of that day, during my more awake moments, wondering if and how I could negotiate my way out of the final evening dose. Fortunately the opportunity didn't arise for me to beg to be let off, as I am sure I would have embarrassed myself. Later that same day when I was feeling horribly sick I decided the natural remedy was a lot better for my body than yet another dose of anti-nausea drugs, so like every good ex-anorexic I went to the bathroom and helped my body to evacuate some of the toxins. I did feel a whole lot better afterwards, and fortunately my face didn't take on the features of a hamster this time, which is just as well as the same Unfavourite Nurse who ignored my symptoms before was on again.

So… I was moved into Iso 2, which is a twin-bedded ward. My last experience in there was horrible and I have tried very hard not to end up there again. My last roommate left the door open when she went to the bathroom, and didn't once flush the toilet or wash her hands. It was revolting and the nurses were horrified when I told them afterwards. When they wanted me to move to Iso 2 this time they promised that the lady sharing was lovely and that I could even choose which bed I wanted to help soften the blow.

Dorothy was indeed truly wonderful. One of those light and gentle beings you feel blessed to have met. She suffered her first bout of cancer about three years ago and was treated on a trial with a new drug. Last year the cancer returned in another more aggressive form, and because of the damage caused to her bone marrow by the first lot of chemo there isn't anything she can be given, so she is on palliative care only.

Stories like this horrify me and are a huge part of my reticence for originally wanting to opt out of chemo. It is fine looking at all the figures and assuming that the bad side effects won't affect you, but when you meet someone who is one of those statistics it is truly shocking. Dorothy was brought in because she had woken up that morning in incredible pain. When you are a chemo/cancer patient Ward 11 is always the first port of call, regardless of the problem. The up side of this is the fabulous care, the down side being that they are cancer experts not any-other-part-of-the-body specialists.

The first day was spent with her lovely husband by her side and an endless stream of blood tests and an attempt to get her pain under control.

What a brave lady. The nurses always ask, "On a scale of 0-10 where 10 is the worst pain in your life, where would you place your pain at the moment?" Judging by what I heard from my side of the room, I would have gone straight for 10, in a 'put me out of it until you have found the problem' kind of way, but no, Dorothy went for a reasonably painful 7. What was she thinking?! I can only think she wasn't really thinking at all or she would surely have gone higher. She even found time to have some gentle conversation with me and to show sympathy for my symptoms, something I found astonishing and almost angelic.

My evening dose arrived bang on time and as there had been no plea bargaining I just had to get on with it, much like the rest of chemo really. My least favourite nurse was on night duty, which made my heart sink. She is gentle but ineffective in a chocolate fireguard kind of way, and takes ages to get anything done. Dorothy had finally fallen asleep so unfortunately the whole procedure of taking me off the drip at midnight woke her up as it went on forever. I felt really sorry for her. I could hear she was awake but she didn't ask for any more pain relief. I managed to drift off to sleep but woke up around 4 in the morning feeling horribly sick. I could hear that Dorothy was asleep and knew that if I called for Unfavourite Nurse it would wake her up and I couldn't do that.

Several people have told me since that I should have done, but I disagree. How on earth can my feeling sick even begin to compare to the level of discomfort this lady was suffering? Did I have any control over my attitude and my body or not? This was the time to find out. I promised myself that if I was still feeling bad in an hour I would hit that buzzer, or at least collar someone when they came to disturb us for water, or blood pressure readings or whatever. Unfavourite Nurse was still on duty an hour later when the water was changed so I asked for some anti-nausea meds, pleased that I had avoided disturbing Dorothy. But in the event I still had to wait 45 minutes for them to appear. Just as well I wasn't in a hurry then.

Just to back track a tiny bit I should say that I had developed a bit of a temperature and a rash the night before. In the middle of all my other woes I wasn't that bothered, but the doctors got over-excited and there were veiled threats of keeping me in for another day. As far as I was concerned, I was going home, rash or no rash. Every time I shivered with a bit of a temperature I threw the duvet off so the icy cold air conditioning could cool me down naturally – and it worked!

I'm delighted to report that come the morning the temperature was gone and the rash had subsided quite a lot. The anti-nausea had helped and I instigated Operation Evacuate. It is amazing how having a higher goal in mind helps one focus on the job in hand. By the time Stephen arrived at 9.30 I was showered and ready to leave. Fenella was packed and all traces of pink had been consigned to my bags. One of my favourite doctors appeared to discharge me and commented that as the flamingo was packed there was obviously no way they were going to keep me there :-). Glad they are learning to read the signs!

It was brilliant to be home, but after a couple of days the rash really took hold. This is a known side-effect of the Cytarabine but by the time I went for my appointment with the consultant the following Monday it was driving me mad. Burning ants scurrying around under my skin is about the closest description I can think of. I tried all kinds of visualisation but was incredibly grateful to come away from my appointment having had an IV injection and clutching a prescription for a course of anti-histamine. I see this as yet another indication of my body rejecting the toxins.

I had another one of those 'AHA!' moments on Monday, thanks to the insight of one of the nurses. I have been taking Olive Leaf Extract again to try and bring my heart under control. I had stopped with the advent of chemo at the stern admonition of one of the nurses, but decided to start again after the last extremely bad interlude when it went out of rhythm. The results so far shall remain unspoken but let's just say I am pleased. So it was with some surprise that I woke on Monday feeling all weak and useless again, only without the palpitations. Not quite as bad as before, but as I was due in for another 1 day chemo treatment (more of that in a mo) I figured we were going to the right place to ask questions. My blood test showed I was neutropenic, and when I mentioned my weakness to the nurse she said it was my body telling me to rest. Haha! That word again! How funny that it keeps cropping up.

With the best will in the world, it is very hard to be positive about the chemo when my body is continually screaming "Noooooooo! Don't do this to me!" and throwing up all kinds of evidence that it is unhappy. But at least the end is in sight. There are a few high fences between me and the finishing line though. The reason I had the additional 1 day chemo (hope you are keeping up with all this) is that on Monday and Tuesday I go in for the stem cell harvest in which my blood is drained out through one arm, filtered through a machine to remove the stem cells for future use, then put back into my body through the other arm with hardly any stem cells and in a potassium, magnesium and calcium depleted form. Lots to look forward to there, then.

The 1 day special earlier this week was a 'purging' just in case there are any cancer cells left. This is where I start to get confused. If all the cancer cells are supposed to be gone, why do I have to have Cycles 5 and 6? This in itself is called into doubt by a slip of the tongue from my lovely consultant. He was curious as to why I got the rash this time but didn't with the first treatment of Cytarabine, and then he said "Well you won't be having any more of those so it isn't a problem." There was all of a two second pause in which I thought 'there's something you're not telling me here', then like a terrier down a rabbit-hole I was on the case with lots of questions like, "That was only Cycle 4, do you mean I don't have to have Cycle 6? And if that is the case, do I actually have to have Cycle 5?" You can imagine. In his endearing, chuckling, Buddha-type fashion he wouldn't be drawn, but clues have been given and I am hopeful in a very cautious kind of way that the finale to this crazy interlude might be slightly differently choreographed to what I was expecting, nay dreading.

The stem cell harvesting experience is going to be interesting for lots of reasons. The stem cell co-ordinator, Lisa, is lovely, but we're not that well acquainted yet and we have to spend 4 intensive hours together. Apparently she is with me for the whole procedure as I can't be left once it has started. I will be unable to move anything except my mouth for four hours so I don't fancy her chances as a willing target for my questions, and I have a few. She was present during our appointment with the consultant on Monday and there were a couple of things that piqued my interest. She mentioned that from my blood results it seemed that whatever I was doing on a dietary/ alternative treatment level is working – which prompted both of them to ask exactly what it is I am doing, but of course it wasn't the time or place to go into details. There will be lots of time on Monday should the topic arise, which I will ensure it will. And secondly she filled out the consent form by hand and has the most spectacularly beautiful handwriting.

We published a book a couple of years ago with Darrelyn Gunzburg, AstroGraphology: The Hidden Link Between Your Horoscope and Your Handwriting. *Whilst I won't get the chance to look at her chart while*

I'm in there, I want to find out what lies beneath such an apparently medical and left brained person. I am sure she has hidden talents and she won't be able to leave my side until I have unearthed some of them. Haha!

This has been a monster blog as there was so much catching up to do. There is loads more too which I will try to include with the stem cell harvest experience. My mum used to tell me how I was christened at the Harvest Festival service of our local church. Let's hope this harvesting is equally calm and fruitful.

And finally, please, please, please go to this link. http://www.youtube. com/watch?v=BaQdwTsVtCY I have already posted it on Facebook so some of you may have seen it, but Megan Kowalewski is inspiration personified. Unfortunately her cancer has returned but she is staying strong. She has bravely posted lots of other videos about her stem cell transplant experience which I will be watching before my own next week.
Wishing you a warm, sunny weekend
Margaret xxxx

During the woes of that very long night in Iso 2, I would have given anything not to have had that final IV bag, the one that goes late into the night. I found it hard to drop off and snooze like a lot of other people did when they were on the drip but something really strange happened for the last half an hour. I fell into a really deep sleep and was only woken when the drip alarm went off. Imagine my surprise when I got this email from Judy the next day:

It was a funny old night. Did you happen to feel like you were dying, or wanted to about, 11.30-11.45 last night? I was doing my breathing machine for my blood pressure and holding a lovely crystal that Terrie and I worked with in Egypt – the one that caused a blue lotus to pop up out of my head. I had already asked Guisseppe [Jeni's guide] to step up the healing for you but I was suddenly whisked off to your bedside and held your hand while you went through the whole weighing of the heart ceremony before Osiris.

Luckily you passed the test and eventually we were ushered out of the underworld into light once more. I've done it with a group before but never as powerfully as this was. It really seemed like you had to make a choice to live or die at the deepest level of your being, and chose life, so no more cancer cells. Does that resonate with what was going on with you?

Er – yes… just a bit! I looked up the Weighing of the Heart ceremony and was a bit shocked – I was pleased I was out for it as it looked really scary. None of these things seem to scare Judy of course. I replied:

The things you are going through for me! Just before that time I was indeed desperate and very low. I was almost ready to beg them not to give me the last session as I felt I really couldn't cope with it, but fortunately for my pride the opportunity didn't present itself.

However, very unusually, I fell deeply asleep during the last half hour, the period of your experience, and was woken up by the machine beeping as the drip had finished. That has never happened before so I wonder if I had to be 'out of it' for the ceremony to take place. I slept fitfully after that as I felt sick and headachey but as the lovely lady I was sharing with had only just got to sleep I didn't want to ring the bell to get medication, so I kept taking myself off to my hammock.

I have to say that is what probably got me to sleep for the ceremony as it seems to be a very powerful visualisation for me… Having just looked at the list of 42 negative confessions, I must have made it through by the skin of my teeth! But why would I go through that now? Is it a choice thing, an initiation? I am fascinated. I have to say that every cycle gets worse as they have a cumulative effect. I was violently sick again and that really takes its toll on my throat – which isn't a good thing. It still hurts today. Although I have only two more to go (apart from a purging one next week before stem cell harvest) those two have grown in proportion to what they were in the beginning as I react more strongly to them and thus they are a lot worse. If this ceremony has giving me some hidden strength that would be wonderful. Presumably (hopefully?) by choosing life my body will cope better. I can see how people get weaker and weaker with each cycle, so it becomes even more important to get really fit in between.

It was humbling to have such support. It felt like my day job was to get as fit and well as possible while all these crazy things were going on in my subconscious.

The good thing about regular blood tests and the constant monitoring is that the medics could swoop in and rescue me if required. The bad thing about blood tests is the psychological hit it gave me when the results weren't so good. We were cautiously planning on going away for a few days before the stem cell harvest to meet our good friends from Preston, Jennifer and Steve. Both had been giving us healing and support from afar, and we were hoping to meet in Glastonbury for a few days. We needed a bit of normality, but normality seemed to have flown out the window when I signed the consent forms.

Red Alert

Blog #22A 19th April, 2013

Good evening lovely people. Back from the hospital and more blood tests in preparation for the harvest on Monday.

Not fabulous news unfortunately: my neutrophil count is a big fat zero, which is as low as it can possibly go. This means I have no immune system whatsoever so am on house arrest as opposed to being taken into Ward 11, where they all know I would be very unhappy. I am lucky to have such understanding doctors. My haemoglobin count is also very low at 81 when ideally it should be over 100.

All of this means the stem cell harvest on Monday might have to be delayed and I will probably have to have a blood transfusion which I really don't want. Can I ask that those of you who have me on your healing list direct the focus to raising both white and red cell counts? I asked once before and the results were astonishing. Thank you so much.

It is strange how these things affect you psychologically. I went in for the appointment feeling slightly tired but generally quite good. Being told that you must stay away from people and be virtually isolated on bed rest definitely takes the bounce out of your step. I am sure there was a little one when I went in, and room for the odd chuckle, but I definitely feel worse now than I did. However, I will be taking myself off to my hammock on the beach (see previous post) for some R&R. I also have a beautiful new purple laptop to play with, which makes it much easier to keep up the blog. Hopefully there won't be such big gaps in communication in future.

Several people have asked about Dot as there hasn't been much mention of her of late. She really is a treasure, and a important part of the incredible nursing care I witnessed last week. I only spent a few hours on the four-bedded ward, but during that time she worked so hard with those ladies to cajole them into eating and drinking. High protein drinks are given to patients unable to eat and she pulled out all the stops, persuading them to choose a flavour then sitting with them for a moment to make sure they had a few sips. She also totally came into her own today. There is about an hour's gap between having the bloods taken and the doctor's appointment to dis-

cuss the results. *During that period I decided to avail myself of the facilities and duly trotted towards the female conveniences.*

Now I have been going to this ward at least once a week since early January, so I am pretty sure I know where the toilets are. *I was about to push the door open and realised it had a great big MALE sign on it. I know I am suffering from a touch of chemo brain but this was strange. I went round the corner to the one that is usually MALE in case there had been some mysterious role reversal, but that was still in its male incarnation. I passed the nursing station towards the next one, which was MALE too. I felt really stupid. Had I unwittingly crossed over into some alternate universe where there were no conveniences for ladies?*

I was standing in this confused state when Dot wandered by, so she asked if I was OK. *I explained the dilemma. She thought it was odd too, and went to the FEMALE lately turned MALE facility and knocked on the door. Nobody in there. She ripped the sign off the door, and hiding on the reverse was FEMALE, so she whacked the sign back on showing the female attribute, and we were home and dry and a lot more comfortable. We both had a good laugh as that was before I got the blood results! See, it's not what you know but who...*

We had a good meeting with Lisa, the stem cell co-ordinator, today. *She was the one to give the blood results too, but she knows how much I hate staying in so it was her involvement which probably got me allowed home. I gather there wouldn't usually be any choice, so I am really grateful for her understanding. She was also telling us more about the process and the machinery involved, which does sound truly amazing. I thought it was going to be a metal machine a bit like an old fashioned tea urn (no idea where that came from!) but you get to see all the blood cells being taken off and separating from the plasma. It sounds much too complicated to explain properly so I am hoping I will be able to video some of it on my phone and of course share with all and sundry.*

Hospital is such a weird mix of science and humanity. *I despair at the way anything perceived as 'alternative' is so often squashed or derided, especially in hospitals, where science is truly king. But these people, these nurses, doctors, technicians, porters, volunteers, cleaners, they really CARE. When I was considering leaving chemo for a while my consultant was really troubled that I could end up being a lot worse off. Some would say that is because he only believes in the science, but that isn't so. He and all the other lovely people I have come into contact with really, really care, and they want their patients to get well and be discharged, permanently. We might have differences in our perspectives and beliefs, but ultimately what matters is that you are surrounded by people with your best interests at heart.*

I have been fortunate enough, up until this illness, to spend very little time in hospital, and I think I was expecting to find a real life portrayal of the worst that is written in the media. The food, clearly, is right up there, but otherwise I couldn't have been more surprised. I was asking one of the nurses today how the blood test samples get down to pathology so quickly, and she replied that there is an army of volunteers who are regularly ferrying notes, samples, whatever is required, between departments, which explains how my file seems to appear magically wherever I am. I have never seen any of these people so they must move like the wind. But it did get me thinking that when I am through all this I would like to help in some way. I'm not really a tea trolley kind of person, but belting between different points in my MBT trainers really does appeal and it would be a fabulous way to get fit as well as give something back to the people who are helping me so much. So now I just have to get well :-).

Wishing you a sunny weekend

Margaret xx

Despite my best attempts I had to go back in for a blood transfusion, which meant we had to cancel our weekend away. Looking back I can't really believe that I thought I would be well enough to go – but maybe that slightly blinkered stubbornness is what kept me going. I emailed to Jennifer:

Sorry don't feel much like talking. So disappointed for lots of reasons but I suppose being very anaemic is causing me to feel that way.

I was so hoping to get through this without reneging on my ideals – good diet and supplements would do it and I wouldn't have to have the transfusions. Then it all went tits up when the chemotherapy-induced anaemia didn't behave like ordinary anaemia, so although they would wait if I insisted on not having the transfusion it seems a bit counter-productive so I have given in. Judy has already lectured me on the necessity of giving up all control and allowing everything to help me that possibly can, but holding on to just a bit helps me to feel less like I am being sucked into a system that might not, in the long run, cure me.

That isn't meant to sound dramatic, but having spent a lot of time on Wards 10 and 11 in the last 2 weeks, all I have seen are people who are in because their cancer is back. Granted, you don't see the successes because they are obviously not in hospital. It is just incredibly depressing and I suppose my resources are low. Fortunately Stephen's aren't, or he is managing to hide it as he is my biggest cheerleader.

Bless her, she replied:

Don't feel guilty about feeling sorry for yourself. Anaemia, as well as having a very debilitating effect can make you feel depressed. With a bit of luck your blood count will soon start to come up again and you will be back to your old cheerful self. I'm glad the platelets have made an improvement.

I can quite understand how coming into contact with people whose cancer has returned isn't exactly helping you to say upbeat. I can only say hang on in there because so many of us are rooting for you and are determined that the treatment is blasting away all the nasties and restoring you to full health.

Like Judy, I did wonder whether you might need to relinquish control of some part of this process as it is occurring under a Neptune transit. I think maybe those of us who are sending healing need to concentrate on you receiving 'good' blood that is free from negative vibes... Obviously there is more to it than that but if everyone works on purifying the blood (physically, emotionally, mentally and spiritually) it will do the trick without damaging you in any other way. We also need to work on lifting your spirits.

This made me feel so much better. Jennifer works on the esoteric level and I knew that she would be sending extra healing my way. How could I not feel more positive? I would periodically apologise for being a bit 'down' in the blogs – but it made me feel good to get the feelings out. This writing business was becoming very cathartic indeed; examining my thoughts as I wrote them into the blogs prompted, and allowed, a lot of introspection.

In on the Action

Blog #23 23rd April, 2013

Ever determined to use the time available to me, I'm typing this from Ward 10 (the Outpatient version of Ward 11) while connected to the IV drip, down which is coursing the irradiated blood from somebody else's veins.

To bring you bang up to date, things went downhill rapidly after my last post. My haemoglobin stubbornly refused to come up despite everything I could throw at it and on Sunday I had to admit defeat and come into Ward 11 for a platelet transfusion. This all happened because around the same time as my white cell count should have been coming up, one of the almost non-existent hair follicles on my leg decided to become infected and turn into a giant blister. When you are neutropenic, the main source of infection is from your own body.

Trust me, you have no idea of the maintenance that goes on overnight in a properly functioning system. Did you ever see the film Westworld? Set in a sort of futuristic Disneyworld, once the punters had left for the day the robots came out and cleared up everything ready for the next influx of excited tourists. The red and white blood cells do the same thing while you sleep, only in my case the workforce is so understaffed there aren't enough to go around. My poor, besieged and debilitated body tried to lob the last few remaining white and red cells at the infection, which not only wasn't enough to help but plunged me into negative everything. I woke up Sunday morning covered in bruises, which is a sign of serious anaemia, so was left with no option but to call the ward, who duly told me to come in so I could have a transfusion of platelets. These are cells that help the blood to clot, and also help the body to repair itself.

This was all very bad news for the stem cell harvest organised for the following day. I went home after the platelets feeling much better but not magnificent. We were due in to Ward 11 the following morning at 8.30 for a pre-harvest blood test, but nobody was really expecting the procedure to go ahead. Bloods were duly taken and the Great Wait for results began. My consultant Joe was in clinic so I knew we would have to wait a while, but there was no decision until 2.30. Yes, 6 hours of doing absolutely nothing.

We had come in expecting to go home almost immediately, so apart from a bit of reading material we were just kicking our heels ALL THAT TIME.

When he finally arrived Joe was really apologetic, but having been on the receiving end of his caring skills, I found it hard to be cross. He said my blood counts were so low I would have to come in the next day for two units of blood then back in again on Wednesday and Thursday for the harvesting. So that's another four consecutive days in hospital. Thank heavens for the free parking!

The whole issue of having blood has been a really big one for me. Psychically speaking I am like a sponge – I have had to consciously work on my boundaries through the years with the result that I am extremely wary about anything being introduced to my system. I have enough problems with what is already there, without taking into account somebody else's 'stuff'.

There was a whole 'ick' factor about the blood and the fact that it has been created in another body that quite probably likes different food from me and has a different lifestyle. After all the care I have taken with my diet, alternative remedies, meditation and visualisation, I could end up with blood from a pizza loving, fizzy drinks swigging person who, although undoubtedly doing their bit by donating blood, could potentially introduce into my body lots of things I try so hard to avoid, plus on a psychic level, a whole lot more.

Of course, by the same token it could be totally pure and of a lot more benefit than what is already in my body (which, quite frankly, is doing a rubbish job). The blood is irradiated, which means it won't have any impurities and I wouldn't actually catch anything, but it still isn't mine… and that troubles me greatly.

Tuesday dawned nice and bright and sunny. The blood transfusion took four and a half hours, so including setting up and the blood test I was on the ward from 10am until 5pm – almost a day's work then! Did I mention before how impressed I am by the care of the nurses and doctors? Just wondered. Today they blew my socks off. You wouldn't think a cancer ward would deal with emergencies, but a whole load came through today and I was in prime position to people watch.

Amongst them was Jean. Do you remember her from one of my earliest blogs? She was my first room-mate and we bonded over our IVs. Absolutely lovely lady who is on palliative care; she has Aplastic Anaemia and can't be cured. She comes in every few weeks for a transfusion and also in between when she gets ill. A slight temperature means an infection, which can become critical in a matter of minutes when you are that ill and we are all reminded relentlessly to call the ward immediately should it happen to us.

The first thing I knew about Jean's arrival was when her wheelchair came past me and was parked next to my bay. I almost didn't recognise her, and it shocked me when I realised who it was. The staff swung into action, firstly to hug her, then get cannulas fitted so she could be wired up to antibiotics and more importantly, saline solution, which really is a life saver. Then a constant stream of staff came to see her and hug her. What really undid me was Dot. She appeared after the cannulas and before the doctors – and cried out "Jean, why are you here again?" then sank to her knees to give her a massive hug, the two of them quietly sobbing together. I don't think there was a dry eye in the place and I was really struggling to hide the tears streaming down my face.

After several chats with the doctors, who were very cross with her (in a loving kind of way) that she waited a whole day of feeling bad before coming in, Jean was sent off for x-rays before being admitted. By this time I had been moved into the bay opposite her so the doctors could pull the curtains round her more easily. I thought she probably wouldn't recognise me as I had hair when we last met, and as she was falling in and out of doziness I didn't want to impose on her, desperate as I was to make contact. However, as her wheelchair was pushed past me on the way to x-ray, Jean lifted her head, gave me a great big smile and said, "You look great, Margaret, just keep on going." I managed to stammer out a completely inadequate, "Get well soon Jean" before they wheeled her away. Cue more tears.

So it has been an emotional day. It is sometimes hard to stay positive in there as, by its very nature, the people that come to Ward 10 are sick – you don't get to see the well people as they don't need to come back. What you do get to see is the tenacity and strength of the human spirit manifested in someone like Jean, who from her tiny and very poorly frame holds high the torch for the rest of us to follow. I would love it if you could include her in your prayers.

Be well

Margaret xxxx

Gulp. Comments came in on the blog as did emails to both me and Stephen; people had quite clearly taken the whole ward to their hearts. This whole experience is bringing out so much emotion, even now as I read the blogs back to put them into the book.

The cancer ward is the sharp end of life, without a doubt; there is something about cancer that strikes fear into the very heart of us. I knew that every patient on the ward was facing, or had faced, the same dark nights and utter terror as me. When I found out that my cancer had a proliferation rate of 90% – obviously very aggressive – I couldn't stop thinking about this thing growing inside me at an alarming rate, and there was a comfort in knowing that I was not alone. To see people like Jean battling on in spite of ever debilitating health was all the inspiration I needed, although there was plenty of it around. There is a tremendous camaraderie in both Wards 10 and 11, where a sick sense of humour and almost war-time spirit prevail, and this really helps the patients to get through the treatment.

Several of the nurses told me they asked to work on these wards – they considered it to be their true calling to be working with such ill people. One of them told me she had deliberately transferred from orthopaedics as she was fed up nursing whingeing footballers in plaster (her words, not mine!). Her attitude was, "Get a grip, you've only broken your leg/arm etc. It's not the end of the world." She had us in fits with her stories. To cap it all she was really pretty and had a wonderful energy about her. She had clearly found her vocation.

It probably sounds weird but I found that once I lost my hair people were really, really nice to me. You wouldn't think there would be any reaction from shop assistants or just people in the street, but it is amazing how many times they would stop to chat or share their journey. Or take extra time to help, like the lady in the health food shop.

We were fairly regular visitors by this point and as my eyebrows were finally going the same way as the rest of my hair, I needed an eyebrow pencil. I'm not the vainest person on the planet by a long stretch, but obviously if in my own view I looked better then I felt better too – not quite so much like a bald little alien. When the hair goes, the follicles do too, so my head was left really shiny and kind of sticky. I expect completely bald men get used to this as they gradually lose their hair, but for me the instant baldness was very strange. So the manageress of the shop took time to find me makeup to suit my newly unadorned state. She was lovely and I really appreciated it. All these little kindnesses add up to create a real feeling of being loved and supported by people you don't even really know.

And so the relentless march of the treatment continued. I still wasn't completely convinced that I wanted or needed the stem cell transplant or its attendant risks. However, Lisa was winning me over by stealth and I had agreed to have the harvest – the transplant was still under question. At least in my mind. The transplant was a truly fabulous experience.

Centrifugal Force - Frankensteina speaks

Blog #23A 24th April, 2013

You will not believe today. In fact you will so not believe it that I have recorded two videos that will go up on YouTube once they are edited.

The whole process of the stem cell harvest depended on my blood test this morning so it was a pretty tense time. The results came back and as my blood cells seemed to be on their best behaviour we were all systems go. I will post a much more detailed description and hopefully attach the video link in the next few days, but suffice to say I was wired up to a machine worthy of Star Trek or Dr Who. The actual wiring up was very painful. It took three attempts to get the cannula into my right arm (the supposedly 'mobile' one) then the left arm, the one that would remain rigid for the next six hours, took a lot of dedicated work by the nurse to offer up its vein. The machine is a new, updated version of the older one, so we also had the benefit of the trainer who was absolutely lovely and was there to teach one of the nurses how it all worked. As it turned out we had many hours at our disposal to communicate with each other and we bonded over our approach to alternative medicine, children and Big Pharma.

More details soon, as I am very tired, but I have to tell you this:

My blood has been taken out of my body through my left arm, pumped through a machine that separates out the plasma, the stem cells, and the red cells (video to follow, amazing, trust me), then returned through my right arm in a reconditioned and cleansed state, not once, but two and a half times. How incredible is that?

And even more importantly, the volume of cells obtained from the harvest is pretty impressive. I asked how many cells they were looking for as I heard that a couple of million would be good. We had to wait an hour for the results to come from the lab, but it was worth it. The nurse told me that to make the maths easier they just deal in single figures. So two equals enough for one transplant, and four would be good (which is what my consultant wants). The result? Nine. Almost as good as Strictly Come Dancing *at its best. So I don't have to go back tomorrow for a rematch and I now have four days ahead of me with no hospital appointments.*

And how I do feel? Amazing. I thought I would be completely exhausted by being rendered immobile on a futuristic machine from 9.00am until 3.00pm but I feel enervated, invigorated and cleansed. I feel better than I have since this whole debacle got underway in January. Thank you from the bottom of my heart to all of you who send healing and are in this for the long haul. This isn't an easy journey and Stephen and I appreciate every single thought and every prayer.
There is a lot more to follow :-)
Margaret xxx

And I really did feel amazing. I felt cleansed at the deepest level and not at all tired from the experience. It was quite hard staying still for six hours and I kept food and drink to a minimum as I didn't want to have to let it out again. There is nothing like being told you can't go to the bathroom to make you need it, is there? Apart from having cannulas in both arms the procedure wasn't really uncomfortable – but watching my blood come out of one arm, go through the machine to have plasma and stem cells extracted and be fed back into my other arm was beyond surreal. I felt incredibly lucky, almost euphoric, while it was going on. I was also lucky that I got on so well with the transplant nurse, Laura, and the rep from the company who own the machine and also provide the training for the nurses. I was attended the whole time as the slightest movement would cause the cannula to move which stopped the blood flow and the machine would spin down.

It was also brilliant to discover that I had several million stem cells waiting to be transplanted, but there was still a question mark over the procedure, at least in my mind. Looking at the statistics, obviously it would improve my chances of survival over a longer period. However, there were huge risks involved. The chemo would be much stronger than I had been given up to this point and there was a very real risk of damage to major organs. There was also the small point that I would be incarcerated in isolation for at least three weeks, and need several months afterwards to recover. Cathy was doing an amazing job of keeping The Wessex Astrologer running in my absence but this was a lot to ask. However, I was feeling much better physically so I was optimistic it would be resolved.

Feeling Good

Blog #24 3rd May, 2013

It's Friday, a Bank holiday weekend, and I'm feeling good! There's a weird, yellow thing in the sky too, which I hear tell is the sun :-)

I was feeling good anyway but I am feeling especially good now as my lovely consultant, Joe, has just phoned with the MRI scan results. I hadn't written a blog this week as there seemed to be so much happening and I was constantly in a state of 'wait-and-see'. So much so that I have just had to delete the paragraph I had written because as of 5 minutes ago when Joe rang it is out of date and I have no idea how to relate the last week as it is all out of context now. A bit like being asked to write a history essay and go backwards and forwards at the same time. Never my strongest point. I'll try not to be too confusing but please do bear with me.

Joe wanted me to have a mid-term MRI scan so he could see whether I needed to have Cycle 6 or not. Cycle 6 is horrible, 3 days of chemo that are long and very hard on the body. If there were no obvious signs left of the cancer then his thinking is that I have a break of about a month after Cycle 5, which is scheduled for next Wednesday, then go into the stem cell transplant on 11th June. More of that in a minute. Just to relieve your no doubt heightened state of anticipation, he called (Friday night at 7.00 — impressive huh?) to tell me that the scan was clear, no sign of anything abnormal. So we can go ahead with Plan A.

Just before all you lovely people start a-whooping with joy that I am cured, I just want to do a very Moon-Pluto in Virgo kind of thing and put this in context. An MRI scan only looks at your body at a tissue/organs kind of level, and certainly at that level it has shown there are no extra weird lumpy bits. Mantle Cell lymphoma is strange in that has the smallest molecules of any of the cancers known to sciencekind. The only way to ascertain whether there is a single molecule left in my system (which is all it would take to start the whole shooting match off again) is to have a PET scan, which is the one where I have to run around all irradiated avoiding pregnant ladies and children. I'm not having one of those just now as my poor system is already rather debilitated and the last thing it needs is ir-

radiating – that could cause a completely different kind of cancer and I do think I have enough to deal with as things stand. I will have a PET scan at the very end of all this. So where are we, exactly? It would be tempting to say that I am in remission, but sitting here with no hair and having lost one-and-a-half-stone in weight with another cycle of chemo scheduled for next week I think that is a bit premature. There is still a very long way to go, and the stem cell transplant is a huge part of that.

You know it is really funny, I was thinking about writing the blog as we drove home from work tonight – I have managed 3 whole days in work this week, I am so proud – and the whole focus has changed just because of that phone call. I was going to write about my day in Ward 11 on Wednesday. I had to go in as a day patient so I could get the MRI scan done early (other-wise it was the end of May), which basically meant I go in and sit next to a bed and pretend that I am staying in order to buck the system. Don't knock it, it works. The rather bizarre bit was that when my time came for the MRI scan a porter turned up with a wheelchair. Apparently it is against Health and Safety regs for a perfectly ambulatory (just learnt that NHS phrase!) and able in-patient to walk themselves anywhere for an appointment – you have to be pushed in a wheelchair.

I was beyond embarrassed. I find it hard enough to be in a wheelchair when I actually need it so you can imagine how this felt. We shared some really bad taste jokes about wheelchair races and I offered to push him when his tea break was due, but the nicest thing was when we were in the lift. Several people got in with us, and amongst them was a very lovely looking lady, slim, elegant, long hair nicely scrunched up. Anyone remember the Boddingtons advert? This lady looked really classy – she opened her mouth and it was pure Essex. I can say that, as I am an Essex girl myself :-)

"Ar long are you in fur luv?"

I replied, big smile on my face, that it was just for the day for a scan, and that I could walk, really, it was just the Health and Safety regs.

She beamed back at me and said "You're doin' great luv. I was in fur free munfs – lawst me hur jus like you, an look at me nah," touching her lovely hair.

For international readers who might not understand that bit, she was saying that she, too lost her hair and was in for 3 months of chemo as an inpatient and she was looking pretty good now! I have to say that heartened me considerably.

One of the most interesting things about this illness is the way my thought processes are changing. The biggest impact, out of all the things I have read, is the Buddhist practice of mindfulness. It is dramatically changing the way I look at each moment, and thus the way I view the world. My world, too. Yes, I hated being in the wheelchair, and the whole scenario, as someone who had driven herself to the hospital and walked into the ward, was completely ridiculous, but if all of that hadn't happened, I wouldn't have bumped into the lovely lady in the lift. I am – finally, some would say, my dear mum included – learning to live in the now, instead of the 'what could be'. Yes, there are lots of things, and people, I would change if I could. But I can't. All I can do is deal with what arises right now, and I am starting to enjoy that process. Every moment is becoming a lot more interesting and exciting as I am emotionally and intellectually present, something that is quite new for me; instead of racing ahead to future opportunities and possibilities, or acting out possible scenarios in my head, I am becoming grounded – albeit very slowly – in the present moment, and you would not believe how good that feels.

But I need to go back to my day on Ward 11 on Wednesday. I pitched up at the nurses' station early in the morning to find out which bed I wasn't going to occupy in order to get my scan. I really can't believe this. There are 16 beds on this ward. Five of them are in isolation, two of which are in my most hated room – the cold, double-bedded Iso 1 and 2. Where was I? Iso 2. I HATE it there. Have I got "I love Iso 2" written on my forehead?

One of my major problems with the stem cell transplant, when I will be in for about four weeks, is that due to the low white cell count I am likely to be in an isolation bed. These beds are in a wing that faces North and have a separate supply of air via a unit which belts out freezing cold air from the vent above the bed. It is not pleasant. I actually find it really depressing, and it was horrible just being there for the day. There is no fresh air, so the constant smell of antiseptic and the other noxious chemicals used to cleanse everything in sight really start to get to me and I find that by the end of my stay – whether it is hours or days, I am gasping for fresh air.

I have the distinct feeling that everybody hates it there. Cancer patients, by their very nature, keep coming back, and I am beginning to suspect that the people who don't shout loud enough end up in Iso 1 and 2. I am extremely troubled by the prospect of a four week stay in hospital. I have bonded

*well with Dot but she can't change the totally revolting food. I really like the
nursing staff who go out of their way to help. But I can't do without fresh
air. I don't care how much the Iso wards protect you, I really can't manage
four weeks on air-conditioned and recycled air. So I might just have to become somebody who can't cope with the cold. I think that might just do it as
the Isolation rooms are all chilly.*

*I realise this is all too much detail and it could be incredibly boring for
some of you, in which case I do apologise, but I feel some forward planning
is necessary. Living in the now is totally wonderful, but I can't help feeling
a little help is needed when it comes to stem cell transplant time. There is so
much more to say but it is Friday night and the weekend starts here! I will
be back with more soon.*
Wishing you all a warm and sunny weekend
Margaret xxxxx

Lovely comments came in from the blog, all of which helped me to
feel so much stronger. It was an amazing feeling to know that other
people in different parts of the world were thinking about me. Dolores Ashcroft-Nowicki is one of my authors and the current Director
of the Mystery School, The Servants of the Light. She sent me this:

Dear Margaret,
*What a lot of lovely news… you sound so much better, all the prayers and
thoughts are coming together. But we must try even harder and not let up
on anything that can help. I just got back from 4 weeks in USA lecturing…
each time we did a ritual I sent some of its energy and power back to you.
You are an inspiration to everyone around you. Love and strength,*
Dolores

Other people, completely unknown to me had also found their way
to the blog. I had this from Joe Tomsic in the US:

*Hi Margaret… please keep it up. It's almost a play by play for me and, ac-
tually, brings back good memories… especially of the great medical people
I met. I'm also a mantle cell survivor having had my stem cell transplant
at Duke in December of 2010. So far so good. Just wanted you to know
that there are others out there who know what all you're going through.*
Joe Tomsic

It was so important to hear from other people who have been through it and are still around to talk about their experience. The comments on the blog were empowering but humbling. It prompted some lovely conversations with Stephen which unfolded over the next few days.

Lazy Days

Blog #25 6th May, 2013

It really has been the most beautiful weekend. We decided not to book any-thing in the diary and to simply take each day as it came, lazy or not. Next week will be frantic, both from a work and chemo perspective, so it was nice to literally 'take a moment'. I love the conversations that arise when we don't have an agenda. When we have the luxury of sitting in the conserva-tory, and as the day wanes, follow each thought to its uninterrupted conclu-sion. How often do we get the chance to do that?

Our thoughts have been turning increasingly to Life After Treatment as the end to this nightmare hopefully starts to edge into view. Every commit-ment, every routine, every dream was unceremoniously dumped when we got the cancer diagnosis; it is such a shock that one's life is turned upside down, and any Grand Plans suddenly become inappropriate in the light of a newly re-arranged and treatment-based schedule. But now there is a strange feeling of being cast adrift at the end of this without a game plan, because we are very different people now from the ones who started out on this journey. It is like being turned, blinking, into bright sunshine after a long time in a dark room – one that I never planned on visiting, as I'm sure nobody does. Even after four months, I still feel as if I was signed up to the wrong club by mistake, and that very soon someone is going to realise I am a fraud. I'm amazed it has lasted this long to be honest.

Stephen and I had a really interesting conversation about this last night, as the light faded and we watched the bats zipping back and forth across the lawn. Some would say I am/was in denial, and they may well be right, be-cause I don't think I have ever really emotionally engaged with this illness, and I have no desire to. Yes, I was shocked to my core, yes, I have felt truly awful (and will do again as I'm not finished yet), yes, in a way I am very frightened about the future, but I have always felt like an imposter on the cancer ward, and I wonder if this is one of the things that has helped me to keep going.

People have said such lovely things about my strength and being an in-spiration (all of which I find it really hard to relate to, but thank you!), but I am beginning to think that the way we cope with illness is programmed into our genes. I hate being ill and have always fought against it. I'm not being brave, I just wake up every morning with a head full of ideas, and sometimes get really cheesed off because I'm not well enough to carry them out. I am much too busy to be ill, and whilst I am very interested in what is going on in my head, the most important thing for me has always to get back into full working order as quickly as possible. And that doesn't necessarily mean 'doing' something. What it does mean is that I don't want to be distracted by being ill. I am equally happy sitting thinking thoughts to myself and pursuing an inner journey as I am editing the next book or packing boxes. This illness has proved very thought provoking and challenging; it has given me something to write about and has brought me unexpected gifts of friendship, love and support that are humbling and beyond my wildest dreams but I am bored now. I want my health back and I have a Lot Of Stuff To Do. And I am quite sure the cancer ward and Dot have a lot more people to be looking after.

Maybe I am just getting itchy feet. My mum would really laugh at that. I didn't exactly have a reputation as a child for sticking with something to the end, and I haven't changed in all these years. With Venus in Gemini the temptation is to skim over the surface of something, then shout "Next!" So yes, I know how horrible and long Cycle 1 is, and I know how gruelling and horribly toxic Cycle 2 can be. I think the stem cell harvesting machine is totally brilliant and I kind of loved that day in a perverse way, but I have had enough now. And I also need to have a really good talk with Joe next week, because I am troubled by the logic of the transplant situation. The week before the stem cell harvest I had a 'purging' session of chemo, which, as the word suggests, was supposed to drive every last cancer cell from my body so that the stem cells harvested would be squeaky clean and untarnished and suitable for transplanting back into my system at a later date. Now that implies, to me, that there was absolutely no chance of one single cancer cell being sucked into that machine. If there was, they would be re-infecting me and I am quite positive that isn't part of the plan. I can understand that my consultant wants me to have Cycle 5 just to be absolutely sure, but what I DEFINITELY don't understand is why I need to have the whole stem cell transplant scenario.

I'll explain the procedure just so you can see where I am coming from here. In four weeks time I will go in for 5 days of extremely toxic and intensive chemo. I have already had very aggressive chemo, but this will be even more noxious and intensive – 5 long days of much more toxic treatment designed to kill off all of my bone marrow. Why? If it was good enough to provide eleven and a half million perfectly formed and untarnished stem cells, why do they want to kill it all off and take me virtually to the point of death?

I really hate management speak but I have to say this doesn't appear to be joined up thinking to me. If it is to any of you, please let me know. So, having taken me to the point of death I will be unceremoniously hauled back to the land of the living via an infusion of the stem cells that were extracted when I was – wait for it – healthy and cancer free. Eventually, after about another 3 weeks of foul hospital food I will supposedly bounce back to life with renewed vigour and be able to leave hospital.

I'm joking about the bouncing back to life. This is a major, major procedure with risks like total kidney and heart failure, so you can understand why I am being extremely circumspect. And I have always had a problem with things I don't understand – it started with maths when I was about 6 and followed through to Physics, Chemistry and Latin. Thankfully English has never been a problem :-). If I don't understand something it really troubles me, and I have to say that the logic of all this is really troubling me. So I will be having words as soon as I can and will report back.

I am very aware that a huge part of my attitude and ability to cope with all this has come from the loving support of many friends – and in fact people I didn't even know but who have taken me to their hearts and sent healing nonetheless. It has come in many forms: I am included on the healing lists of prayer groups and healing circles around the world. Dear friends have had pujas said for me in Indian temples and Greek monasteries, and I know I have been included in the healing rituals of many different religions and beliefs. The stories I have had back from some of these merit a whole blog of their own, and hopefully I will be relate these in due course. I'd like to take a few lines to tell you about one such experience which has been going on as a kind of 'back story'.

My dear friend and author Judy Hall had a holiday booked to Egypt which departed in early February, a couple of weeks after my first chemo treatment. Judy has been visiting Egypt for decades and she wanted to take a photo of Stephen and me with her so she could ask the gods for some *healing for us. This also coincided with the arrival of the box of pink hats, so Judy came over to take a photo of us modelling them – and it was this photo which was taken around Egypt, literally. We were taken up the Nile and participated in many trips into temples and tombs and were also presented to mummified crocodiles as well as being laid gently in the wings of Isis and surrounded by a healing mandala of stones created by Judy's cabin steward.*

Stephen and I somehow became part of the whole journey made by Judy and her friends as our photo was taken from one sacred site to the next. My healing became a sub-text of their holiday. I can't even begin to do this justice so you need to go to Judy's website judyhall.co.uk and download the pdf account of her time in Egypt which describes in detail the sites she visited and the history and mythology behind them. I just feel incredibly lucky to have been in the presence of such powerful entities, and I know their influence and healing continue.

A busy old week now so I will be in touch when I can. Blood tests and the doctor tomorrow then that lovely long 12-hour day hooked up to the chemo on Wednesday.

Enjoy your week!

Mxx

Researching your own illness can be a double-edged sword. When you are right in the middle of treatment it isn't good to read the downside of it and, especially with the stem cell transplant, how toxic it is. I was really worried about surviving the toxicity and getting my health back afterwards; this is where the internet and the blog is so wonderful. Yes, I had access to the more unpalatable side of the treatment, but I also found a huge amount of support. I found a few stories from cancer survivors who had come through the transplant, and they gave me a huge amount of support. I realised I was at the very edges of scientific advances in having this treatment, and I knew that I had to be up to the job both physically and mentally. Daunting stuff, but much worse of course when it was residing in my head instead of being made manifest in hospital.

Dolores was right there with a comment that warmed the cockles of my heart with this:

Dear Margaret,
You continue to amaze me with your determination to win through this
ordeal and get your health back on form. You are an inspiration to us all.
Having just got back from the USA I was shattered to find I had less than a
week to unpack, get my sleeping patterns back to normal, repack, and print
out 4 x 34 rituals for the coming weekend workshop in Manchester...Little
old ladies of 84 are usually watching daytime TV and knitting socks!! Not
careering around the countryside teaching Magic!!
But then I think of you and it gives me energy and strength to get up and
go... Bless you dear.
lots of love
Dolores

Thinking of me was giving her strength! That was amazing and I
admire her energy. Joe Tomsic came back with this lovely inspiration
and advice for me:

Hi Margaret... really appreciate your writings. You're going to do very,
very good with your treatments and bone marrow stem cell transplant. I
was first diagnosed with the mantle cell lymphoma in April of 2010 and,
as I mentioned in my email, had the bone marrow stem cell transplant in
December of 2010. I'm doing great and you will, too. Unfortunately, and
unlike you, I didn't do anything special as far as diet in preparation for the
transplant. Your preparations should enhance the entire process for you.
*   I asked the doctors at Duke, after the 'regular' chemo program in my*
hometown, to take me as low as they could... and they did. If I could offer
any advice it would be to try to eat during the four weeks of treatments
prior to the procedure. I couldn't and eventually told the nurses to stop
bringing the food. Thank God for the IV food. The other thing is try to
force yourself to walk... even if a little. Just walk the corridor with your IV
stand. They'll also tell you to go directly to the hospital if your temperature
goes up. I tried to do exactly as they instructed in all respects. I have the
most fantastic wife in the world and she was there every inch of the way
doing everything for me. It was actually tougher on her than it was for me.
As far as follow up treatment, I'm on an every other month Rituximab IV
treatment. It takes about two hours and there are little to no side effects.
Strictly maintenance and maybe something your doctors might recommend.

I know almost exactly what you've been through to date and what you're facing. You're going to do really, really great and you're going to be so proud of yourself. Your results will be even better than mine. The bone marrow stem cell transplant is going to do it for you. The most important part of all, however, will be the prayers you are, and will be, receiving.

Guess what. I just received an invitation to the Duke Survivors dinner. So there you go. By the way, you're already an inspiration. Best wishes Margaret.

This was just what I needed to hear. Onwards! Unbeknown to me, my uplifted mood was also somewhat accounted for by the drugs I was on. I like to think there is an 'up' side to most things, and I have said previously that the medical staff do all they can to make you comfortable during the treatment. One unexpected bonus to all this was the steroid element of the treatment. Steroids are given to help the lessen body's reaction to the chemo in some of in some of the cycles. I didn't realise they would have more of an effect on some cycles than others.

Steroid Heaven

Blog #26 10th May, 2013

Didn't expect to see that title for Cycle 5, did you, huh?

The totally excellent thing about Cycles 1, 3 and 5 is that for reasons I can't remember due to chemo brain (an excuse I find I am resorting to a lot now) I am given five days of very high steroid treatment immediately after it. A bit like after childbirth where the (supposedly) wonderful event of producing the child blanks out the pain blah, blah, blah (sorry but it didn't work that way for me), so do the highs of steroid heaven make you forget the horrors of the chemo. So just before I completely forget I want to tell you it was just as awful as before only slightly more so.

I would say that ignorance is a wonderful thing when it comes to chemo, because as the cycles go on, your mind, and thus your body, start to act in a similar way as your pet does when it knows it is going to the vets. You only have to get the pet carrier out and They Know. And it is also like the game 'I went to the shop and I bought'. Uh huh. Your body knows exactly what it bought last time and it has no intention of going back for more.

On Cycle 1 I was all gung-ho, wide eyed and 'Let's get on with it chaps', at which the nurses smiled winningly, knowing how it would all change later down the line. A horrible experience to be sure, but no sickness. A lot of tiredness and discontent at how long it all took, but pretty good considering. Cycle 3 took even longer = even more grumpy plus violent sickness. The morning of Cycle 5 came and without any conscious intention from me whatsoever, my body had backed into the furthest corner from the pet carrier. I dragged it unwillingly to the hospital, and would you believe it, despite all attempts to the contrary my chemo wasn't ready so we STILL couldn't get started early.

This cycle has lots of different components and the last part is three sessions of a wonderful drug called Mesna which is to protect your bladder and kidneys from the searingly destructive effects of the rest of the chemo. These doses have to be given three hours apart with a saline flush in between, so with that plus all the other stuff it is a horribly long day. However, this time I had secret information which would help me avoid an overnight stay and thus an even longer incarceration. It was a little confusing, but it did work out in the end, with quite a lot of added benefits. I went in as a day patient, which theoretically meant I should have been in Ward 10, which is nice and bright and busy and I love it there. But there wasn't any space on Ward 10 so I was booked into a bed on Ward 11 but with my own nurse, one of the stem cell transplant team – she was available as there was no transplanting to be done that day. I don't really like Ward 11 much as by contrast it is quiet, cold and airless in that very special way that only double-cycled air conditioning can create. Imagine my surprise when I was shepherded not to my usual and much-hated Iso 2 bed, but whisked through another door to the stem cell transplant suites. Wow. Never knew about this!

I was shown down this secret corridor, that I swear never existed before, into a room that has its own bathroom, fridge, television, dvd and cd player, exercise bike, steps for more exercise and windows that look over a grassy area and that appear to OPEN. Oh and a huge squishy chair that reclines and has a fancy footrest that comes up too. Premier Inns eat your heart out.

The chemo did eventually get started and I settled into my des res ready for the Long Day. Several advantages presented themselves almost immediately and my rather wobbly and indecisive attitude to the transplant started to become slightly more positive. This magical Harry Potteresque corridor seems to house a few cupboards and fridges itself, which equals gatherings of people which equals gossip. The very first thing I learnt was the lady in the next door suite had asked if she could please not have scrambled eggs on toast for breakfast tomorrow. What? Is there more to life than Readibrek á la NHS? Dot goes to these cupboards a lot so she also came in to chat a lot, always a bonus. She offered me a cup of tea and as I had forgotten my stash from home I asked if she had any herbal tea. She didn't, but managed to snaffle some green tea from the staff cupboard which is also there. How handy is that?!

When my designated chemo nurse came in we got talking about such breakfasts and in the process I found out that on Day 1 of the transplant schedule I have a chat with the Dietician. Oh Goody. I really cannot wait to see what the NHS idea is of a good healthy diet to recover from the five intensive days of chemo that are required pre-stem cell transplant. Apparently it is her say-so as to whether I can have a cooked breakfast and other goodies, so I hope she has set aside a goooooooood long time for a chat. She can also 'advise' about supplements and vitamins, so anything I can get on the NHS instead of taking out a small mortgage for at the health food shop would be good, but on the other hand it had better BE good – none of your replicant Big Pharma ideas of vitamins and supplements.

I am so excited. Do you think she will be ready for a frank and open discussion about the benefits of Aloe Vera Juice in preventing nausea, plus the effects of all the other stuff I am taking? I do hope so. Because, you see, my nurse and I continued to have a very enlightening discussion that included the benefits of yoga, meditation, and especially the fact that due to the exceptionally fine advice I was given right at the beginning (thank you Swamiji and Manisha), the Vitamin A drops have completely stopped me having any of the mouth problems associated with chemo, as has the linseed tea prevented any buildup at the – erm – other end. Something which is apparently also an issue judging by the huge amount of bottles and pills I was sent home with to deal with the problem. I know, from what she said, that my case is exceptional, so THIS STUFF WORKS. Anything I can do to see this information included in advice given out to future patients would be absolutely wonderful. So, I am afraid the Dietician is in for quite a session because if she even starts to try and utter that phrase about the science not supporting it she is going to be in trouble.

All of this was very stimulating and very exciting. I also found out the answer to my stem cell question before I made a fool of myself in front of Joe. The stem cells taken off at harvesting time are wee babies which haven't become red, white, lymph or anything yet. They are pure as the driven snow and their only mission is to imbed themselves in the bone marrow and thus create a new me. Totally, from what I gather, as every other cell will be totally annihilated during the preceding five days of chemo. Apparently only mature cells can become cancerous – although I am going to check this at my appointment on Monday – which is why it is safe to put back the stem cells. All very incredible really.

None of which detracts from how horrible Cycle 5 was. It was exceedingly long drawn out for the reasons stated above, and we finally got finished at 10.30pm. Which is whole lot better than either 12.30am or 3.30am, which it was before but it did involve me being violently sick again at the end and repeating the hamster look-alike act. This time I didn't say anything about *it as I knew it would delay us even further. The nurse discharging me did ask if I was very tired and I just said I was and slunk out the door. Probably a bit naughty but my need to get home was pretty intense by that time.*

When we did get home I collapsed into a pretty blissful and uninterrupted sleep which I would never in a million years have got in hospital and felt a lot better for it. Except for my face of course. My eyes were swollen so much I could hardly see out of them and my chin and neck had become one solid pillar of flesh. Lunchtime approached and I finally called the ward to check it out – previously they gave me anti-histamines for it so I wouldn't have minded going back in for a shot of that. The lovely doctor just suggested I stay at home and take paracetamol as it would probably go down on its own. And indeed it did. So today I am high on steroids and feeling fine. I'm so sorry if this blog has tired you out. I realise there is quite a belt of energy in it which probably means that I need to slow down and take it easy tomorrow. Unlikely but I will do my best.

Wishing you a splendid weekend wherever you are

Margaret xxx

Although Cycle 5 was undoubtedly horrible, I was in much better spirits regarding the transplant than previously. I got the distinct feeling that the long period in hospital that it required would be a different experience from my other incarcerations – for one thing the transplant suites were a lot more welcoming, if any hospital room can be – and additions like a fridge and an ensuite bathroom were really important. Only later in the process would I understand the need for the ensuite! It would give me that little bit of independence that is so vital in these situations. My conversations with the nurse during Cycle 5 were also encouraging; it was good to have some support on the ward for my interest in alternative therapies, and she gave me the courage to be more open with the other staff. It is very easy to see the nurses just as people doing a job which happens to involve doling out very toxic chemicals, and forget that they have their own lives and interests – many of which, it would transpire, were similar to mine. Yes. After an astoundingly negative attitude to the transplant at the outset of treatment, I was feeling a lot more positive. However, I still had a few weeks to go, and my thoughts were, as ever, on physically surviving the whole process.

Sunday Roast Post

Blog #27 12th May, 2013

It only struck me as I named this post how synchronous were my thoughts with the Christchurch Food Festival, which is a lovely community event running in our local town this week. We went down yesterday just before the rain hit and really enjoyed wandering amongst the, generally, good quality foodie tents and soaking up the ambience. It was lovely and a pleasant change from hospital and resting.

My last post generated quite a few blog comments and emails about food and diet, so rather than try and answer people separately I thought it would be easier to do a Sunday Roast Post. I'd like to clear up a few things before we get started lest you think I have turned into some paragon of virtue who spends her hours perusing a wide selection of lettuce leaves as she sips green tea. Oh no. I still have a taste for and thoroughly enjoy the odd glass of Chardonnay and yesterday had a totally decadent slice of Banoffee cheesecake.

I did manage several weeks as a replicant bunny, straight after the visit to the herbalist, but being so strict was beginning to take away the little bit of enjoyment I was managing to have in amongst the hospital trips; I found that mealtimes were becoming something almost to dread so I am slightly more relaxed in my approach than I was, but still pretty vigilant. I have chosen to follow a very low carb diet with a lot more veg than meat because that it what suits me. I don't like the effect that carbs have on my body and I don't miss them in the slightest – to me they are just fillers for the real stuff. But that is moving away from what I really want to say. This post has been the hardest of any of them to write – it would be so easy to get up on any number of the soapboxes I have lined up here, but I don't want to do that as they are mine and I am very protective of them. You have to find your own. This whole blog is about MY voyage of discovery.

It matters a huge amount to me that the food I put into my body is as good as it could possibly be. I constantly bear in mind a conversation with Swamiji many years ago when the whole obesity/food quality crisis was just beginning. Her thought was that our bodies are not satisfied with nutri-

tionally deficient food and thus they crave more. If the vegetables we eat are grown from suspect or GM seeds on mineral deficient soil with the aid of fertilizers, or in the case of animals, reared in a horrible great shed with no daylight, fresh air or proper food, how can they possibly in turn be doing us any good? Whoops, one of the soapboxes crept out there!

But truly, this is a journey for all of us. Those of you who have asked questions need to go off and do your own research. Trust me, it is empowering. If you have an underlying medical problem, especially if it is chronic, become your own expert. The wonderful thing about the internet is that you can do all your own research without moving from your home or paying people a fortune for their advice, although of course sometimes it is good to go and talk to a professional in your chosen area of research. Find others who are struggling with the same condition and learn from them. Research the treatments that have helped them and come to your own conclusions then push it further. I go by the rule of three, which I discovered in astrology but I am sure exists elsewhere – once I have read something three times in different places I give it that bit more credence and follow it with more interest (as long as it isn't just copied and pasted from the same source). And make sure it is up to date. I scared the life out of myself that first morning in hospital by following old links to mantle cell lymphoma. Even two years ago it was considered incurable with a very short life expectancy, but new research from earlier this year shows that my regime may hold the possibility of a cure. Check, check, check your data, and don't base your knowledge on biased Big Pharma-funded scientific trials or clever marketing. It is only by talking to people and reading that you get to amass your own arsenal.

I am incredibly lucky in that I have several people around me that I trust implicitly with my wellbeing. They have loved and supported me through the hardest times in my life and they have absolutely been there for me in these last few, very trying months. Find your own support team. You don't need hundreds of friends, each having their own opinion and draining your energy. Appreciate and listen to the ones who count and who are in it for the long haul – they are the diamonds.

I think it is also really important to be flexible and move on from things that are no longer appropriate or don't work. It doesn't matter how far you go down a particular route – what matters is that you have been open enough to explore it. I have decided not to pursue the Oxygen Therapy as I noticed some changes in my body I wasn't happy about. I am also taking a break from the ayurveda for a while as I don't feel it is appropriate right now, but either of these are open to review in the future. What matters is that you constantly question and push and keep your own agenda in mind.

Here's a brilliant example (promise no soapboxes). The chemotherapy is taking its toll on the condition of my skin, which is now very dry and looking like it should belong to someone a lot older than me. I take Omega oils every day as well as vitamin A and D drops, add Jojoba oil to the bath and regularly moisturise my skin, but it isn't enough.

We were in our very favourite local health food shop yesterday and asked for some advice. The manager recommended coconut oil, which I remember using on my hair years ago... really weird stuff. She said it is better than vitamin E (which is what I went in planning to buy) and given that you can use one massive tub for lots of things we thought we would give it a go. I don't want to venture into strange territory here, but you can cook with it, smear it on your skin and eat the stuff. The possibilities are endless. I also added a few chunks to my bath, which of course immediately dissolved and created a lovely oily mess but the results were amazing and I am (at the moment!) a convert.

So go, explore, read, listen and constantly question, with an open mind and an open heart.
Be well,
Margaret xx

A period of relative calm followed, with the exception of some hospital visits and a trip to the local restaurant which ended with me belting my head on the taxi door... which of course took me back to hospital again.

...And on the Seventh Day

Blog #28 22nd May, 2013

God, grant me the serenity to accept the things I cannot change,
The courage to change the things I can,
And the wisdom to know the difference.

This blog seems to have a life of its own – I really do just feel like the messenger sometimes. I had some ideas on Sunday which were forming into something interesting, then finally started to write this last night, but didn't finish. As I come to it today (Wednesday) there is yet more that wants to come out, mostly media related.

Did any of you catch the Radio 4 programme about cancer and diet? It was interesting, but sadly just confirmed that there is actually no proper dietary advice for patients and it is all as bad as I thought it was. The consultant interviewed was really supportive of the concept but he admitted that he spends all his time keeping up to date with the latest developments in chemotherapy and with the best will in the world doesn't have time to advise on diet, even if he knew anything useful. Which of course he doesn't because nobody in the NHS is willing to step outside the 'science is God' framework and consider for a moment that diet can at the very least help recovery from the ravages of treatment. So, as we all suspected, it really officially is left to the patients and their loved ones to do the research. Obviously a gap in the market here. Which brings me to the next sound bite.

Maurice Saatchi was on the Radio 2's Jeremy Vine show yesterday talking about his wife's death. She suffered from ovarian cancer but died through illness related to the toxicity of the chemo she was given and the resulting debilitation to her system. Something which you know is very close to my heart as I approach with some trepidation my own stem cell transplant (more of that below). It is good to have such a high profile and articulate person involved in fighting the battle against cancer. Why? Because the battle isn't really against the cancer, which at the moment, with an estimated 1 in 2 people being diagnosed with it, is winning hands down; it is a battle against a system which provides no protection for those brave souls who are trying to cure it. For anyone confused and surprised by that statement, I will explain.

My frustration expressed in the paragraph above comes from the unwillingness (understandably) of the medical profession to step outside what is scientifically proven. This unwillingness comes from the knowledge that, in law, if they suggest something to a patient which deviates from accepted protocol and that patient consequently dies, then they can be sued for negligence. If, however, the patient follows an accepted course of chemotherapy and dies from the toxic side effects or infections, it is recorded as death from the cancer.

Which is of course untrue.

Maurice Saatchi has requested a Medical Innovation Bill to be passed in the House of Lords which in effect protects the medical profession from such action. As he so rightly points out, innovation is deviation from the norm, and if deviation is discouraged due to the law, there will be no progress in the search for a cure for cancer. Nobody will try anything radically different.

A massive step in the right direction and one I support wholeheartedly. You can read more about it in the Huffington Post article here
http://www.huffingtonpost.com/2013/03/13/maurice-saatchi-wife-ovarian-cancer-bill-experimental-therapies_n_2867353.html.

Hopefully Lord Saatchi's endeavours will also lead him towards questioning the stranglehold and bully-boy tactics of Big Pharma which currently subdue any opposition to them from alternative therapies.

I was doing a bit of research of my own at the weekend. I have found that about 12 days after treatment I get a really sick and sore tummy plus a feeling of weakness. The cells in the stomach, gut and mouth replicate fastest, so this is where you first notice problems – there is nothing to replace them once they die off as the baby cells that were growing in my bone marrow were killed off in the last bout of chemo and the new ones are only just being created. Vitamin A does a huge amount to alleviate mouth problems, hence so far, no ulcers or thrush, but my stomach starts to feel really raw. I discovered that L-Glutamine is an amino acid, effectively one of the building blocks of the body, and you can take it as a powder, dissolved in water. It is especially useful for stomach problems. Sounds like a chemo patient's best kept secret! Forgive my rather basic scientific approach – you can go look up all the long names if you really want to.

We wandered rather slowly (I wasn't having a good day) to our favourite health food shop where the lovely assistant explained a lot more and confirmed that lots of chemo patients use it. I couldn't help thinking, 'Well, Duh! It would have been nice if someone could have told me about this several cycles ago!' You know sometimes it is the most incredible hard work being ill and I do get irritated that these products are available out there but the short sightedness of the healthcare system precludes any truly useful information being given out. So instead they just throw you some more pills. Anyhow, got the powder, miraculous recovery in, oh, about 2 hours I'd say. So anybody out there who is suffering, go and get some nice white L-Glutamine powder to put in your water.

Monday came and with it our appointment with Joe to discuss the Big Plan. Yes, there is no Cycle 6, yay, but he painted a pretty bleak picture of the stem cell transplant. We did have a good laugh though and there was a moment when he looked a teeny bit scared of us and slightly bewildered. He said that there are in fact 6 days of very harsh chemo (not 5 as I previously thought), so, wait for it, on the 7th day... I get the stem cells.

The symbolism (and possibly strain) was all a bit much so Stephen and I just looked at each other and burst out laughing. We were cracking all kinds of bad jokes about me being recreated on the 7th day ... and on the 7th day I will rise again, as you can imagine. Or maybe you just had to be there. Order was restored after a few minutes and we concentrated on the fact that the chemo will definitely kill all the cancer cells that week because it will more or less kill me in the process. There won't be a single bone marrow cell left standing amidst the rubble of my body after all the drugs have done their work and that is a really scary thought.

It is incredible what they can do these days. But it is also a sobering thought in that they will be rebuilding me from scratch by putting back about three quarters of the eleven and a half million cells they harvested a month ago. As you can imagine, this is going to be very hard work for my poor body so Joe said I should expect to feel pretty bad in the week following chemo.

Cue L-Glutamine, Vit A, Vit D, wheatgrass protein, turmeric, Aloe Vera and anything else I can muster. I told him about all of these and he is more than happy for me to take anything that might help. Just as well as I was going to take it anyway. Although I quite possibly have the most amazing consultant in the world I do get tetchy when other methods of support are ever so slightly disparaged. Bear in mind that I was still in shock from finding out I would be taken to the point of death and then rebuilt on the 7th day – so I did say that it wasn't just luck that I hadn't had the mouth ulcers, thrush, diarrhoea, constipation, etc. that he always asks me about. It is because I have put a lot of effort into staying as well as I possibly can; thus I am hoping to cope a lot better than expected after the ravages of the transplant.

The issue of rebirth is interesting and we spent a while talking about that – obviously only in the scientific, physical sense as we were after all in the hospital with an NHS consultant. What he said is that they don't know what caused the original cell to mutate. Science has made wonderful strides and in cracking the DNA code has produced a huge wealth of information, but in a sense it is all too much – they don't know how to find specific details within all this so it will take a lot of time to unravel; he is very hopeful that in the not-too-far-distant future chemo will be very old hat and that there will be entirely new ways of dealing with and targeting specific cells. But that isn't possible just now.

So we talked about the possibility of the cancer returning, which takes us into the whole deliberately confusing world of statistics. There is a 70% chance of me still being in remission in five years' time. Which of course means there is a 30% chance of it coming back. It also means that the data is quite new and the odds might be better when reviewed in ten years. What do we do when we are faced with such information, which is, on a personal level absolutely meaningless? I have no idea which group I am likely to fall into, and all I can do is load the odds in my favour of it being the bigger one by taking advantage of everything that comes my way. Stephen and I are coping with all this whole experience by dealing with each day as it arises, and after a few moments of sombre contemplation we decided that the statistics do not form part of this mindful practice.

The conversation between the three of us moved to allogeneic transplant, which is a stem cell transplant coming from a tissue matched donor. The thinking behind this is that my own stem cells, new and pretty as they may be, also carry within them the programming for mutation, so in one sense all we are doing next month is putting back several million cells which I originally made – just one of which could contain within it the potential to mutate. You could go crazy with all this. Someone who is cancer free (currently!) won't carry that potential. However, the risks involved in allogeneic transplant are massive and I don't even want to think about it. What cost regrowth and rebirth? I have no idea but it opens all kinds of cans of worms and my can opener is somewhat over-subscribed at present. That one can just sit there for a bit.

My feeling from the last few days is that I have been through the mill on all levels: philosophical, physical and metaphysical. I was in hospital yesterday for an unscheduled stopover as I banged my head badly on Monday night. We had gone out for the first time in months to celebrate a forthcoming treatment-free period (how the gods love to laugh) and as I had miscalculated my ability to walk to and from the restaurant we got a taxi home. Although I'm not neutropenic or anaemic (hurrah!) my platelets are very low which means there is a risk of bleeding internally from bruising. Whacking your head on the taxi door after a night out at the local curry house more than amply qualifies for concern so yesterday I spent four hours in Ward 10 having more blood tests and a CT scan. Which came back fine BTW. I was on my own in there as Stephen finally escaped to London on a long-overdue visit – at my insistence, poor guy – and he hadn't even got off the train the other end before I was back in hospital. I didn't feel like reading as my head was hurting, so I spent all that time people-watching. And sadly, amongst the people I watched, was my lovely friend Jean, who was brought in by ambulance. She cannot be much longer for this world and it grieves me deeply. It grieves me that there are extremely unconventional treatments out there, like cannabis oil, which are very controversial and illegal, but by which she could still be saved. But she won't be because it isn't being offered.

Do there have to be two worlds? Are they getting closer together? Why does it have to be a showdown between conventional and 'alternative' treatments? How can we embrace the best of both so that more people survive? Surely rescuing more people from the clutches of cancer is way above money and politics. Hence my offering of the Serenity Prayer – if there is any way I can make a difference in all this, I will.

With love

Margaret xx

Big words, written when I was in the middle of treatment and incensed by what I saw going on around me. What I realised as time went on is that it takes such a huge amount of energy to be an agent of change, and I needed to conserve my energy for myself. It was heartening, however, to be able to spread the word at every opportunity – rebellion on a small scale against a system which is heavily biased towards tradition and Big Pharma. My own experience with cancer seems to encourage other people to talk about theirs too, often newly diagnosed, and thus the usefulness of complementary therapies and diet can spread. I was at a loose end after Cycle 5, which was constructive on many levels as it gave me time to get strong enough for the transplant and to ponder the meaning of it all.

An In-Betweenie

Blog #29 1st June, 2013

> *My heart is so small*
> *it's almost invisible.*
> *How can You place*
> *such big sorrows in it?*
> *"Look," He answered,*
> *"your eyes are even smaller,*
> *yet they behold the world."*
>
> *Rumi*

It is strange being an in-betweenie. For the last five months of my treatment there has been a regular rhythm to the cycles: chemo, crawl back to health, recovery of bounciness, next cycle.

I was in Ward 10 on Thursday for the usual blood tests and chat with the house doctor (one of my favourites) and she didn't even wait for the results of the blood tests – and that has happened twice now. Looking at the results of last week's test she said I looked fine and that I was free to go until next Monday when I see my (wonderful) consultant for the pre-stem cell transplant appointment, and after that I will be free for a further week until the chemo and transplant itself. I did a little jump for joy then wandered out into the dreary drizzle of our British Spring.

The jump for joy was quickly followed by the realisation that I have become quite institutionalised since January. I have all my bits of paper sorted out now, I know all the staff by name and they know me, they even know when I am next in and what for, which is all a bit spooky – how does that work? They all asked if my head was better (see last post) which was kind of sweet, but a little disconcerting. I find it hard to recognise faces and remember names – although I am very good with voices on the phone – but they seem to know everyone and remember everything about them. I guess it comes with the territory. All of this brought me to thinking how strange it will be when I get to the end of the chemo and am free to roam the world again. Actually it is quite scary. And where do I fit in? Although I still think I signed up to the wrong club by mistake, I have become used to telling people I have cancer and trotting out all the gory details on request. The treatment schedule and hospital visits have completely taken over our lives and hopefully, after July, a sense of freedom will return, but we are very different people now. After the transplant I should definitely be in remission. I think I will have a PET scan to confirm it, but my head and heart are going to take a long time to catch up. So will my hair. And so will my stamina, which could take up to a year to get back to normal levels, if it does at all.

What I have come to realise is that you can't go through an experience like this, get the (hopefully) all clear, then bounce back to life as if nothing happened – and this thought has been weighing very heavily on my mind in the last few days. I think this is where Stephen and I really get to grips with the whole concept of 'living with cancer' as we maybe haven't before. Assuming everything goes to plan with the transplant, I will return for fewer and fewer visits to the hospital until I am only poking my nose in there every six months or so. Or maybe even yearly. That would be nice. But how do we cope, in that quiet gap between the visits, with the possibility that the dark invader has returned? I can hear you shouting, "You can't think like that!" and you are probably right. But it is very hard to stop those thoughts and also to know how to approach my life now.

I have to say I am writing after three very powerful eclipses, which in astrological terms have given my chart a good beating, so this introspection is not a surprise. I can now understand the deeper meaning of the phrase 'cancer survivor'. I used to think, 'Wow, well done you! Through it and out the other side, and long may your healthy life continue', but I now see it is because, initially, people like me need somewhere to place ourselves, even if it is only for our own benefit. It is so similar to grief. People were lovely to me after my parents died, but after a few weeks most of them went back to normal. I, on the other hand was only just beginning the process of grieving and probably needed more support than ever before; likewise with cancer.

Going through the treatment has been a psychological and spiritual struggle just as much as it has been a physical one, and I have had masses of support to help me through it. Life after the chemo will be different and it will no doubt bring struggles of a different kind – the thought of it already is. My hair will grow back and hopefully my normal level of fitness will return, but my life will never be the same again, and the last few days have been filled with a lot of sadness at that realisation – there will always be fear, at the slightest twinge, that the cancer is back. And I am finding that really hard to cope with.

I had a long conversation with my dear Swamiji, who can always be relied on to tell it like it is. She comes out with the harshest truths in such a lovely, loving voice; the words explode in your heart then the tears come, then you realise just how right she is. I have threatened to publish a book of her wisdom and fully intend to carry it out so that everyone can share the tears and the torment it causes. :-).

Because that's what the spiritual path is. It wasn't something I deliberately chose, but it appears to be something I have been following for some decades and it gets extremely tough at times. Swamiji said that suffering is life's way of keeping us alert to our path. If everything was easy, our souls would go to sleep and there would be no progress.

I personally find that option incredibly attractive just now. As Rumi said, in a lighter quote, "Listen; there's a hell of a good universe next door: let's go!" If there was a bus leaving now, I would be first in that queue. As I can't see the bus stop just yet, I find myself remembering something I said at the beginning of all this: that I couldn't control the outcome of any of this, but the one thing I can control is my attitude. It felt hard work then and it feels like hard work now, but I also believe that out of all the hard work will come reward.

Swamiji also talked about how suffering stimulates creativity. We are forced to dig deep and find ways of coping, and for me (who in the past has felt as creative as a brick), it has taken the form of writing this blog. I have often been asked, as a publisher, when I would be writing my own book, and I have always said that I am much better at working with other people to bring their words into print. I never felt I had anything to say before, but now I do. I have always believed that when you are brave enough to bring worries into the light they become easier to deal with, and I am fortunate in having some wonderful people who encourage me to do so and who are stable enough to support me through the process. Although writing this blog is a bit like washing your dirty linen in public, it seems to be finding its niche. I have been told that some people are finding it helpful and that it encourages conversations with loved ones that wouldn't otherwise have taken place. Splendid. In the cheeriest and most positive way possible, I am *delighted that I can continue to inflict you with my woes. As a great fan of Rumi, let's finish with another of his gems:*

> *Sit, be still, and listen*
> *because you're drunk*
> *and we're at*
> *the edge of the roof*

Enjoy your weekend!
Margaret xxx

I love Rumi and it turned out there were other fans out there too, in particular the multi-talented and very lovely Mario Reading. He came back with this:

I thought you might like to read my translation of Rumi's Ode, Margaret. I agree with you wholeheartedly about the significance of suffering and the importance of acceptance.
See if you like this!
Lots of love
Mario xx

> *What can be done, O believers, as I no longer recognize myself?*
> *I'm neither a Christian nor a Jew, a Magian or a Moslem.*
>
> *I'm neither of the East nor West; of land or sea;*
> *I don't belong to nature; nor to the stars in the sky.*
>
> *I'm not of the earth, or water, or air, or fire;*
> *I'm neither of Heaven, nor the dust from this carpet.*
>
> *I'm not from India, China, Bulgaria or Saqsin;*
> *Nor from the kingdom of Iraq, or Khorasan.*
>
> *I'm not from this world, or the next, from Paradise or Hell;*
> *I'm not of Adam's seed, or Eve's, from Eden or Rizwan.*
>
> *My place is placeless, my traces traceless;*
> *I'm neither body nor soul, as I belong to the soul of my Beloved.*

I have no need of duality, as I have seen two worlds as One.
The One I seek; the One I know, the One I see, the One I call

He is the first and the last, the outward and the inward,
I know no other than He – there is only Him.

Love's cup intoxicates me as both worlds slip from my hands.
My only business now is drinking and merrymaking.

If once in my life I shared a moment without you,
From that moment on I would repent of my own life.

If once in this world I earned a moment with you,
I'd trample both worlds in a triumphal dance.

O Shams of Tabriz, I'm so drunk in this world – now
Only stories of carousal and revelry pass my lips.

I asked Mario if I could use this in my book and he said:

Of course you can. I used it at the end of my book The Third Antichrist. *I used my translation of an Ibn Al Arabi poem at the beginning. How can one possibly compete with those two topping and tailing you!!*

I was finding that if I let people in they would give me inspiration every step of the way and the Rumi-wagon had a fair few passengers by now. He had such a way with words. Sorry, but I have to just quote this again:

Sit, be still, and listen
because you're drunk
and we're at
the edge of the roof

It makes me chuckle every time. Sitting at the edge of anything can be terrifying, especially if you are contemplating leaping over it. There is a whole world of emotion wrapped up in those few words: it is like he is saying, "Listen. *Listen!!* Do you realise just how important all this is?" And mostly we don't.

However, the wheels of the treatment schedule ground slowly onwards, bringing me closer to what I knew was going to be a massive upheaval. At least with the chemo cycles I was only in for a few days at a time – the thought of spending so many weeks in hospital for the stem cell transplant was utterly depressing. Separation is a curious thing. Stephen and I are the kind of couple who like to be together as much as possible. He works for Watkins Mind, Body, Spirit magazine from his desk in my office – the wonders of the modern age mean he can be based down here in Bournemouth but be in constant contact with the shop. This means we are together virtually 24/7, something that would send many couples screaming to the four corners of the earth. But it works for us and we gain much strength from our togetherness. Apart from the horrible food, and worry about work, as Cathy would be completely running the show for a couple of months, I was deeply upset at being away from Stephen for so long. In the same way that 'quality time' with the kids is usually anything but, visiting time in hospital is quite stressful in some ways and very unlike just hanging out together, which is what we do so well. There was a lot going on in my head and my heart as we faced this final hurdle.

Signing My Life Away

Blog #30 4th June, 2013

I have to apologise in advance (and, it seems, retrospectively) for the strain of slightly sick humour that runs through these blogs; I blame it all on my family, as my father started it and it was more than ably continued by my brothers, so you could say it is in my genes. That's my excuse and I'm sticking to it, but it does serve its purpose.

There are particular situations where humour is a very necessary release from unbearable tension. For instance, some 20 years ago we were gathered at our parents' house. Our Mum had died three weeks previously and our Dad wanted to have a little family service in the garden to plant a rose bush in her honour. Unfortunately he was taken ill very shortly after the ceremony and then died at home of a heart attack the following day, which also happened to be Mother's Day. We were all clustered downstairs waiting for the undertaker to come (the same one who had handled our Mum's funeral) not really sure what to do with ourselves as we were all very much in shock. One of my brothers suddenly said, "You could say that to lose one parent is unfortunate, but to lose both could be construed as carelessness." After a second to take in the enormity of the words, we burst out laughing and that really broke the ice. There were loads of sick jokes after that – like asking the undertaker if he could give us a discount for bulk purchase, ditto the florist... it goes on. Sick, but you need it. You can't carry on at such a pitch without something giving.

I had a moment like that yesterday. We had a pre-Stem Cell Transplant appointment with Joe which was, to put it frankly, incredibly depressing. He needed to go through all the drugs I will be given during the six days of intensive chemo and their possible side effects. Don't we love that one? The good old litigation lawyers have made it so you have to be told absolutely every single thing about the treatment so you can't then sue the NHS if there are 'complications'. And I hate them for it. It is bad enough that I have to go through all this without having all the negative side effects (and I have enough of a struggle with those anyway, as you know) written out in full; the process can't help but eat away at the careful cloak of positivity that months of hard work and introspection have wrapped around me for protection. (Why a cloak? Because underneath I confess to feeling scared and vulnerable. But having it protects me while I grow strong.)

Liver damage? Yep, no problem. Kidney failure resulting in the need for dialysis? Absolutely! Sepsis (blood poisoning) leading to life threatening conditions – need Intensive Care for that one. Of course! Wondered what the food was like up there anyway! Heart failure which might result in a stay in the Cardiac Unit? Bring it on.

Having read through all the information and listened closely while it was all explained, I was then shown the dotted line on which to sign. And then it happened. My lovely consultant knows me by now so he started chuckling as soon as the words were out of my mouth. "This is it – I really am signing my life away, literally, like never before, aren't I? Signing a mortgage form has absolutely nothing on this!"

And it is true. The whole thing about consent forms is ridiculous. I have been in Ward 10, busily having bloods taken or whatever, while other people have been given their chemo. When a new patient comes in the nurse giving the treatment has to read through all the side effects and get the patient to sign the form, just as I did. Only some of these patients are not the full ticket due to their age, and also probably because by their appearance they have been round the chemo wheel several times already and are back in with yet another relapse.

I saw a lovely old guy, completely deaf, being prepared for his treatment. The nurse had the form ready. "I just need to go through the side effects with you so you can sign the form, then we can get going." Blank look. "I just need to go through the side effects with you so you can sign the form, then we can get going." Still blank. "I NEED TO READ YOU SOMETHING SO YOU CAN SIGN THE FORM." A flicker of understanding. "THIS DRUG MIGHT MAKE YOU SICK." He nods. "IT COULD ALSO GIVE YOU HEART FAILURE." He nods. "AND YOUR KIDNEYS MIGHT FAIL." He nods. "CAN YOU SIGN THE FORM NOW?" He nods and smiles and duly signs. "NO PROBLEM, LOVE."

Did he understand? Possibly not. Are the NHS and Big Pharma off the hook? Absolutely.

I had assumed that my appointment yesterday was going to be a really quick "see you next Tuesday" affair, but there were reams of paperwork to *complete and a whole battery of tests to be done before I go in. This battery of tests should have been done during the last week but a 'communication breakdown' meant that none of the requests were filled and I wasn't called to any appointments.*

So far from having some hospital-free time until the stem cell transplant I am more than adequately having every day filled by round robin visits to most of the hospital departments. We had to leave our appointment with Joe mid-stream to go up for a heart trace. Some hurried phone calls from the assisting nurse had resulted in "please go up now they are waiting for you", which was probably a blessing for the posse of patients outside still waiting for their appointment. We returned some minutes later clutching the resulting printout, jumped the queue and duly received the paperwork for more blood tests and a chest x-ray, all of which I did today. I also saw Joe again so I could sign another form to waive all the rights to my poor body. He was in a reflective mood today. Yesterday's meeting was sort of manic and there were a lot of people in the room. Him, me, Stephen, student nurse, stem cell transplant organiser, so there was a lot of laughter and the opportunity to fool around for an audience. More bad humour to relieve the tension.

Today was different, just him and me. I signed his form with a sigh and passed it back. He was very thoughtful. He said, really gently, that if there was another option he would use it. He said that in the circumstances the risks were very much outweighed by the benefits. He also pointed out that the benefit and objective of all this is to achieve a long term remission, not a cure. Gulp. I knew that, I just hated him for saying it, but of course he had to. Then he said that when I have been in remission for ten years he will call it a cure, all with a big smile on his face. This man really knows how to get inside my head.

On Thursday I am going for a lung function test which sounds exciting as I have never had one of those. I am hoping that the years of yoga and meditation and watching the breath will have paid off and that they will discover I have splendid and enviable lung function. I think I am free until the transplant then, which will be nice. There is just a teeny shadow on the horizon of an otherwise very sunny day. My blood tests show that my platelets aren't recovering very fast and they have to be at a certain level before the transplant can go ahead. He isn't sure why that is. I am taking folic acid to hurry the process along and will also be eating an awful lot of lamb's liver before I go in, but if the platelets are still low on Tuesday I will have to have a bone marrow biopsy to find out why. This is an incredibly painful procedure which I really do not want. I don't want it because it hurts, but I also don't want it because I don't want there to be anything wrong that we don't already know about. Any spare moments you have to send healing thoughts with this in mind would be very welcome.

And tomorrow? There has been no mention of tomorrow. This is because our wonderful friend Crispin has offered us his beach hut for the day and we're not going anywhere near the hospital. SO happy. Except that I only found out yesterday that I can't sit in the sun (after a whole weekend of sitting in the garden!) because my skin is extra photosensitive due to the chemo. And I won't be able to sit in it for another six months, so there goes the cruise... :-(. But every cloud has a silver lining – at least I will be able to sit by the beach, all tucked up in the shade, just relaxing and reading some seriously good chick lit. Which is about all my brain can cope with just now.

Big hugs to you all,
Mxx

It was in school term time so we were anticipating a quiet day at what is often a very busy beach. There was a beautiful clear sky, a wide, empty beach, and comfy sun loungers to slump into instead of the stones and sand we usually have to put up with. Lovely empty beach until the two ladies with about ten children between them set up camp RIGHT in front of us, about 20 feet in front of the beach hut. Why us? No steps, no toilet, no café, no ice cream kiosk in sight. Just us, trying to have a quiet day out. This always seems to happen to me. Stephen didn't believe me until he experienced it – time and again there will be loads of space, or seats, around us, and people will come and sit almost as close as they can. It is a measure of my fragile state of mind that I wanted to go and scream at them to go away. Fortunately common sense and Stephen prevailed and I didn't. As it happened the children were very well behaved and we didn't really notice they were there after a while.

The day after the beach I went for my lung function test, which was a huge amount of fun as there were lots of different machines to blow into and quite a lot of holding my breath. You can tell how narrow my life had become! I was delighted that the years of yoga etc. had indeed paid off as apparently my lungs are extremely big. An average sized pair of lungs are between 80–120 somethings (forgotten what exactly!) and mine are a whopping 148 somethings. SO pleased. Nice and big and strong to withstand the ravages of the chemo, which is what they were worried about.

I thought I was all lined up for a peaceful few days which would include a visit from my brother and his family, but unbeknown to me, my wonderful team of consultants and specialists were discussing me behind closed doors. All was not well in Camp Cahill.

Making the Gods Laugh

Blog #31 10th June, 2013

The best way to make the gods laugh is definitely to make plans. Or even a plan, especially when you are going through chemo.

We completely cleared the diary when all this started, taking everything very much as it came along, as we never knew what might crop up that would involve a visit to the hospital. That spontaneity can in itself get a bit boring sometimes, and it can also make life a bit difficult. My brother and his family wanted to come and see us before the transplant date; this was quite tricky to organise given my hospital appointments and their far-flung living arrangements and shift patterns, but organise it we did. I was really looking forward to seeing them and to enjoying a few final days before the transplant without going to the hospital. For some reason my emotions in the last couple of weeks have been very up and down – well mostly down, to be honest. The spectre of the transplant and its attendant risks and discomfort had reached gargantuan and unmanageable proportions in my mind, aided and abetted by all the forms I had to sign to show that I knew just how horrible and risky it would be. I was finding it very hard to be positive and my normal bounciness had bounced elsewhere. Spending three out of four days last week at the hospital in what was supposed to be my appointment-free time didn't help matters either. I was low, grey and extremely fed up, but very much looking forward to the family visit.

We were literally just walking out the door on Friday, off to get the party food, when the phone rang. It was Catherine, the Macmillan nurse, saying that at a team meeting that morning (touching that they were talking about me!) it had been decided that I should have another blood test before the transplant to check that my platelets were coming back up. Today. Nooooooooooooooooooo!

I told her that we were literally off to the shops to buy food for our guests who were already on their way to us. She replied that they really wanted to do it today and the nurses on Ward 10 were all ready for me. How can you say no? They all have this amazing way of making you feel like the world revolves around you and all of this is for your own good. Which it is of course, but not on your only hospital-free day when you are preparing lunch for seven people. Grrrr.

I said I would come but could I just have the blood test then zip out again – they could call me if there was a problem.

"Well, the doctors do want a quick chat after the results come back."

This would mean a wait of at least 45 minutes on top of the blood test time and the car journey there and back. It was starting to look like a seriously late lunch. Hurried phone call to my brother. Fortunately Number Two son had blessed us with his presence so we did at least have someone to let them in if we weren't back.

Bloods duly taken, we waited patiently for the results; Catherine came to get us for the 'chat', and I did notice she wasn't clutching the usual paperwork. Hmmm. We all sat down and she prepared the ground, reminding me that the fabulous and ever-attentive Joe, along with his equally wonderful team, were worried by my blood results. This wasn't looking good from where I was sitting. These latest results weren't any better than the last lot and the team needed to find out why. And the only way to find out why? A bone marrow biopsy. Now. Doctor primed, ready and waiting. Again, Noooooooooooooooooooooooooo!

My only day to do something for me, and all this happens! At that point, I really did wonder how much more miserable I could get. I couldn't think of a single funny thing to say, which isn't at all like me. Readers of blog 30 will know how much I didn't want the biopsy as it is incredibly painful and it isn't at all the thing to do as a precursor to greeting a houseful of guests. I tried feebly to get out of it, but Catherine skilfully countered every argument. At her suggestion our lunch menu changed from chicken breasts stuffed with mozzarella and basil, wrapped in parma ham, to French sticks and rolls served with a selection of ham and cheese and salad. Stephen was despatched to Tesco while I underwent the procedure.

There were two slightly more cheery points that quickly became apparent: Number One, it was my favourite doctor and Number Two I was offered gas and air, which I wasn't when I had this done before. This isn't at all the same gas and air I had when my boys were born twenty years ago. Oh no. This was twenty-first century gas and air that blew my socks off.

Needless to say I made very good use of it and was just starting to get lightheaded when Catherine said I should give it a break as I would start to become lightheaded. Oh. I thought that was the whole point :-). Then she said that if I didn't stop I could risk an Out Of Body Experience. I laughed out loud. "And your problem is?... Right now that is exactly what I want!"

General hilarity all round, which took my mind off what was going on. And I'm not going to tell you what is involved. If you want to find out more go and Google it for the gory details. It isn't nice and I really don't want to have another one ever, but at least the gas and air gave us a laugh and took the edge off things.

Procedure over, Joe called by and that is when it got a bit serious, although he said it all with a smile on his face. He started out by saying that the team had decided on the blood test and biopsy and he knew how unpopular it would be with me. That was the general laughter bit. Then he said that there could be two reasons why the platelet count was low: one was that I had had a lot of chemo in a short period of time and that my system was taking a while to recover. That was fine and if it was the case the transplant would go ahead next week. The other possibility was that the bone marrow was permanently damaged by the chemo. This would be very bad. The only way out of that scenario would be a bone marrow transplant from someone else – which carries a 40% fatality rate – or blood transfusions every few weeks for the rest of my life. Which wouldn't, I gather, in all probability, be that long. Definitely not the information to take to a family party. Gulp.

My Family Friday had gone really pear-shaped in the space of a few hours. He said that he would take the samples to the lab and call me as soon as he had looked at them, either later that day or Saturday morning. Poor guy. He was off on a family holiday the same day. Bet that was popular with the family.

Anyhow, we took ourselves home and really did have a lovely time with the family. Nobody minded in the least that their lunch had transmogrified into a bit of a Ploughmans, and a good time was had by all. The evening passed with no phone call and come Saturday morning I was practising Mindfulness like crazy. The funny thing is that, although I had spent all morning quite a long way from the phone, it happened to ring on one of the few times I was passing it, so my hardworking consultant probably thought I was literally sitting on it. Anyway, all good. Platelets are clearly a bit tired by all this but are otherwise fine. There is also no sign of Mantle Cell, which is great. There wasn't originally so I would have been very distressed if some had crept into the bone marrow while we weren't looking. So all systems go for Tuesday.

But you know the weirdest thing about this – and we aren't done by a long shot yet – is that before Friday happened I was dreading next week, and feeling very sad and negative about it. Now – I am delighted! I am well enough to go through the whole thing, as opposed to being much sicker than when I started out. Thank heavens for that!

There is more. You may remember from previous blogs that my dearest friend Judy Hall had taken our photograph on holiday with her to Egypt, so that she could take us to visit the temples of the gods who would help my healing process. Both her connection with the gods and the healing continued when she came back and while I was going through Cycle 4 she went through the Egyptian Death and Rebirth ritual, the Weighing of the Heart, on my behalf. I was deeply grateful that she had done this, a ritual which Imhotep (High Priest of the Sun god Ra), had told her was vital to the success of the stem cell transplant. Last week, however, Judy said that I needed to go through the ritual myself; there had to be an etheric cleansing and rebirth as well as the physical regenesis I will get from the transplant in hospital. This really bothered me. I was tired, fed up and very negative about the transplant when she gave me the news. I have done plenty of regressions and journeys into the Interlife, and a lot of them are emotional and exhausting. I seriously worried that I didn't have the resources to cope. But then Friday came and went, and the relief at the good result lifted my spirits immensely – I decided to go ahead.

Judy said I didn't need to prepare in advance – it was important that I take each stage as it came without any preconceptions. She came over for the afternoon to guide me through it and after a few moments to relax and deepen my level of awareness, I was slowly taken through eleven gates. At each gate I had to lay down or give up something: starting with my clothes and moving through my personality, my past, my family and loved ones, ending with my Self.

It felt amazing. Far from being frightening, the opportunity to give all this up was deeply liberating. And as I have no hair at the moment, I really did feel like an Initiate. I was more than ready for this and welcomed the chance to move into a new life. At the twelfth gate I was taken to meet Anubis (the jackal headed god associated with the afterlife) and witness my heart being weighed against the feather of Maat (the concept of truth, justice and law). I knew little about the whole ritual before I started, but I had heard about the weighing of the heart. It sounded as scary as being judged by your life flashing before you at the entrance to the pearly gates.

Whether you believe all this or not, it is still a scary thought that you might someday be judged on the decisions you have made in your life. I needn't have worried. I was allowed to see that during my life there had been times when I acted out of fear, sadness, maybe ignorance or frustration, but never malice. That was a big relief. It was an opportunity to forgive myself and release the burden of guilt I had been carrying for so long. I felt truly cleansed and moved joyfully through the rest of the ritual, in which I was given the chance to awaken to a new consciousness.

An experience I had approached with a degree of apprehension turned out to be one of the most liberating and beautiful rituals I have ever undertaken, and I am deeply grateful to Judy for guiding me through it. There are some things in life we have to do alone. We have to find the courage to face the unknown and trust that we will not be found wanting. I am being forced to do this on a physical level through the cancer and chemo; on an esoteric level, the shedding of different layers as I progressed through the ritual allowed me to bare my soul, and to discard years of accumulated baggage. It is so hard to describe, but I feel cleansed and liberated and ready to face whatever the transplant procedure throws at me.

Tomorrow the pink camel train starts up again as I gather Fenella, my duvet cover, towels, toilet bag and all the associated clutter needed for a long hospital stay, and this one will indeed be long. Six days of chemo followed by stem cell transplant, then several weeks of crawling back to health before I can plan my escape. This time I'm adding a cafetiere and milk so at least I can have a decent cup of coffee! I will be in touch as and when I can.
Wishing you all good health,
Margaret xxx

I was still bathing in the golden light of the ritual when I got this from Judy:

Dearest Margaret
It was a privilege to walk through the Duat alongside such a light, lovely and courageous soul. How could you ever doubt that your heart would pass

the test? You give so much joy to everyone. I have no doubt at all that you will safely make the same journey now through the physical level of this incredible experience into renewed life. Regenesis – becoming Isis. A true initiate you represent wisdom, immortality, life, fertility and knowledge for us all. You are an inspiration.
Heal well
Mega hugs to you and Stephen
Judy

Crikey. My Virgo Moon was working overtime to keep my feet on the ground with all this loveliness around. And Mario sent this:

This was a wonderful post, Margaret. And a beautiful description of the Weighing of the Heart you did with Judy. In other terms, perhaps, one might call it a Making of the Soul. As they have long been unable to cure my own so-called cancer, I am off tomorrow to be inducted as a guinea pig in some esoteric vaccine trial the Royal Marsden are conducting, in which, I believe, I am to be turned into a bird (or something of that ilk, via fowlpest). A sort of staving off of the evil day. With my luck, I shall probably get the placebo and cause enormous mirth as I claim a miracle cure. Joking apart, as you and I both know, we are not ill. We are simply in a different place. I am hoping, of course, that the bird I turn into will be a Phoenix!! You, of course, are already soaring high, and I have a very strong conviction that you will get through this, just as I did with my first terminal cancer 21 years ago. The sound of God laughing is a beautiful sound.

And I replied:

Hi Mario,
Thank you for your beautifully crafted comment. I see you as an inspiration and someone who is already soaring with the eagles. It would be the best and most extreme irony if you were in the placebo group and made a miraculous recovery.
Thinking of you
Mxx

What a guy. I wanted to include these beautiful comments to show just how vital it is to be supported – to not feel alone. I couldn't ever feel down for very long because there were always some really good, strong, and above all honest people to talk to when the need arose, as it did frequently. I could talk about my fears or whatever was in my head and I knew they would answer me from their hearts. The staff on the wards were like that too: no holds barred and that's what I needed. The whole 'baring my soul' part of writing the blog was bearing fruit in ways I had never imagined.

And so the camel train did indeed gear up the next morning. But not without tears – surprisingly this time from Stephen rather than me. I was doing my best to keep a cheery front despite my heart breaking at the thought of leaving him to be in hospital for anything up to a month. The long months of stress and worry were finally breaking through Stephen's immense strength, and my absolute rock in all of this needed to just cry it all out. It did a lot to clear the air. Obviously one doesn't go around crying all the time, but I think there comes a time when you do just need to cry, and cling together, and admit you are scared as hell and don't have the energy to carry on. Then, having done so, have a final hug, wipe your eyes… and carry on. And that is what we did. Once I was all checked in and Stephen went off to work, it all became much easier and more like a normal treatment cycle. In fact the next week went by in a flash.

Stem Cells Safely Back Home

Blog #32 18th June, 2013

It is done! The build-up of the last six months has culminated in an extremely civilised affair which began at 3.03pm in Bournemouth, today, and included a steaming cauldron containing my stem cells. How symbolic and alchemical is that? I mentioned this earlier to the Wrong Doctor, when she described the forthcoming procedure, and her comment was that she didn't think that Lisa, the stem cell co-ordinator, would like to be thought of as a white witch. She was so wrong. The lovely Lisa and I had a good old chat about it and apparently one of the transfusion co-ordinators really is a white witch. Haha. Lovely. It never fails to amaze me that there exist, within the very staid and politically correct NHS, such diverse and gifted souls who bring a touch of their own magic to the healing process. To be brutally honest though, it wasn't actually a cauldron, more of a grey bin.

Lisa took the lid off and the freezing mist crept over the edges of the bin, just like out of a Disney cartoon. (Did you see **Brave***? Astounding. Hope my hair grows back like that.) Then, using a small tank filled with warm water, she warmed up the bags containing my precious stem cells and attached them to the IV line one by one. Seven million stem cells (some have been kept back as there were originally eleven and a half million). It was so strange to think back to when that was done, and what a huge thing it was. I do have to say – and this is with no irony or hidden agenda – that science is truly amazing. It just gets a bit up itself sometimes.*

The whole thing started last Tuesday, when I was admitted. The only procedure that day was a Pentamidine Nebuliser, which I didn't know about, as I hadn't read the transplant leaflet I had been given. I tried to wriggle out of it of course, as the chemicals used are so noxious that the room has to be sealed for two hours after it is used. You can understand my reticence. If it is that bad why do I have to breathe it in?! I discovered it is to protect the lining of the lungs from a nasty type of pneumonia, and I have to agree it would be silly to go through all this then be seriously ill with pneumonia. I will have to have it once a month for the next six months. So I gave in gracefully. The next few days passed in a haze of chemo and the most intensive nursing I have experienced to date. My previous cycles had nothing on this. It is absolutely crucial that with this level of chemo the bodily functions are monitored constantly, especially the fluids. The kidneys are flushed via continuous saline bags through the IV (at night as well), the objective being to get rid of all the chemo before the stem cells arrive. I have to keep count of all the drinks and use a bedpan so they can measure what comes out. Too much information? Sorry. I lost all my embarrassment on that score way back, when I had the boys!

One of the hardest things about all this hasn't been the physical intrusion and drugs, it is the feeling of never having a moment's peace. There is a really sweet chapel here, and I thought if I could only get there I could at least enjoy a few moments of quiet contemplation. I mentioned this to one of the nurses and she agreed that constant interruptions are the most frequent complaint from patients. She said I couldn't go to the chapel as various alarms were due to go off on my drips and there were more procedures due, but that we could pick a suitable time slot and she would stick a 'Do Not Disturb' note on my door. Result. I had 20 precious minutes of mindfulness practice and emerged refreshed and ready to continue in a much more grounded state. It should be much calmer from now on, so as I still have the notice, I plan on using it every day.

We also used the sign when Judy came to give me some healing, in conjunction with Imhotep. The noise of the ward continued outside, but at least the request for peace was respected. She brought with her a massive chunk of green calcite for me to hold during the process as it is good for nausea, along with a smaller piece for the bedside cabinet. As it turns out, Fenella has become guardian of both, and she is doing a splendid job of leaning against one and keeping a beady eye on the other. For company she also has a carved scarab beetle, a memento from Judy's trip to Egypt. Judy also brought some lovely scented bath bombs. More of them later.

The dietician never materialised as apparently I have to be malnourished before she gets involved. You seriously couldn't make this up. However, Dot has given me access to the Special Menu for patients who can't choose from the regular one for various reasons. I chose an omelette with ham and a bit of cheese for lunch today and wondered if anything edible would arrive. Dot arrived, excitedly bearing the platter on high, and triumphantly delivered it to the office I have established for myself in my room. I took a picture of this – office, not omelette - and only then noticed that the window frame is pink, matching beautifully with my own personal colour scheme. I honestly had nothing to do with that, but I do think the colour co-ordination is a good sign.

I was astounded. This was a really good omelette. It tasted like it was made in a completely different kitchen from the one where they cook the other stuff. Dot returned and was delighted to see, for the first time, an empty plate. Wow. Stephen has been doing a fabulous job of bringing me in home cooked food, so it is good to know that at least he can have a break from it occasionally and know that I won't starve. At this stage it is survival techniques. As soon as I get home I can get back to the diet I really need to be eating, but I do at least have the fridge stuffed with smoothies.

The weirdest day of all was yesterday (Monday – Day 1). Four of the previous five days were pretty gruelling chemo. The days are counted backwards to the big Zero, the day the stem cells are returned, after which you go into positive numbers. All a bit weird. Day 7 was the nebuliser, Day 6 was a quickie half-an-hour chemo session, Days 5 to 2 were a lot tougher, with two half-hour doses of my old friend Cytarabine (10 in the morning and 10 at night), which previously brought up the rash and made me very sick (and did so again this time), and four hours of Etoposide during the day.

At the beginning of the week the days seemed to stretch ahead interminably, and I wondered how I would get through them. I was especially worried about the sickness, but the staff managed it fantastically and I was fine. Day 1 was apparently the 'bomb' in comparison to the other chemo, and it was non-stop from the moment I woke up, but none of it was unpleasant. You probably won't believe this but the worst bit was the ice lollies. This particular drug, Melphalan, destroys the digestive gut from the mouth right to the exit point, and as coldness helps to protect the cells in the mouth I was given ice lollies to suck and crunch, from 20 minutes before the chemo, all the time it was running, then 20 minutes afterwards. Yuk. I hate ice lollies. I crunched my way through two orange Callipos, two mini-milks, a Rocket and a Fruit Pastille lolly, all before noon. I felt so sick, and it has taken until now for my teeth to recover from the onslaught of the noxious chemicals that make up these things.

It is hard to believe I have been here a week, bearing in mind my escape tactics of previous treatments. I have had some amazing conversations with the nurses, and I am sure there will be more, as I am only about a third of *the way through my stay here – the rest of the time being recovery. My impression is that people in caring professions never think they are doing a good enough job. Several of the nurses here have told me they wish they had more time to talk with patients, and although that would be good in an ideal world, I'm not so sure that is where the magic is necessarily transferred from nurse to patient. It is in the daily encounters, the smiling collection of yet another bedpan, the few moments of contact during routine procedures, that as patients we get the sense that someone is doing this job because they really, really want to, and that feels amazing.*

Day Zero has been really nice. With half an hour to spare before the ward rounds this morning, I ran a hot bath. I chose the rose bomb, and was delighted as the water became beautifully oily, scented – and with floating rose petals! As I sank into the water, still attached to the drip, I realised just how bizarre the whole situation was – but it was only later I appreciated that I was unwittingly undertaking a ritual cleansing in preparation for the transplant.

And now, at the end of the day, I am still feeling good. It wasn't as traumatic as I was warned it could be, but I know the days ahead will be tough, as my red cells, white cells, neutropenes and platelets drop. I should start to surface about a week to ten days from now, as my body starts to rebuild itself, so don't worry if there is radio silence for a while. Obviously that is a worst case scenario and I am planning on being back in action much faster than that! There will be much news on my return.

Wishing you well

Margaret xx

There was radio silence through the next two weeks. Immediately after the transplant I felt fine, almost on a high as the Deed Had Been Done and I was out the other side of it. In my usual optimistic way I was expecting to zip through the next few days and be out of hospital in record time. Unfortunately, with the best will in the world, this wasn't going to be the case. At Day 3 after the transplant I was found to be neutropenic so was confined to my room until further notice. Even fresh air was deemed to be too high risk, which seemed unbelievable to me. Then the sickness started.

It was greatly exacerbated by the hospital 'smell' which seemed to exude from my very pores. I wanted to throw up as soon as I smelt the food trolley arrive on the ward, and even my specially prepared Readibrek went back almost untouched. The nurses have an almost limitless supply of anti-emetics to help with the sickness – in fact to help with anything – and you only have to ask. They all come with side-effects though, some of which are downright scary. One of them in particular, Domperidone, made me feel like there were a load of different vices in my head. I am quite happy with my own company and like to be in silence most of the time, that silence being internal as well as external, but this drug appeared to have invited a whole horde of not very nice characters into my head. Needless to say I only tried that once. Metoclopramide gave me bad headaches and ran out very quickly – way before the four hours required between doses. I was offered and tried so many that I forgot the rest of the names. Once the sickness gets a hold it is much harder to control, so I was offered a subcutaneous pump which would allow small amounts of the drug into my system on a regular basis. This seemed to work quite well, but it had to be removed after five days due to the risk of infection. The other massive side effect of the Melphalin is di-arrhoea, and it starts about five to seven days after transplant. Once it started I had to give a sample to the nurses so they could check it wasn't the result of a bug. Having been duly checked, I was allowed Immodium, which made me much more comfortable.

All of this was taking a massive toll on my body. There were three days when I only moved off my bed to go to the bathroom. I could only sleep on my left side as the anti-emetic pump was attached to my right arm. I was dehydrated through not eating and not wanting to drink even water, so I was also on fluids, which were going down the IV into my Hickman line. I didn't want to eat and I didn't really want any visitors. There were a couple of times when I didn't even want to see Stephen, so deep was my discomfort and lack of energy. It was during this time my old war wound of a frozen shoulder reared its ugly head again. The Hickman line had made movement more and more difficult during the preceding months as every time I moved my right arm it disturbed the exit point of the line, which would then get sore – so basically I just about stopped using my right arm for anything much at all. It was already getting achy by the time I went in for the transplant, and the three days of miserable immobility in my bed really allowed it to let rip. Much like the way it announced its arrival many years ago, I went from 'discomfort' to raging pain in a few minutes. It was late at night and I was suddenly in so much pain I had to rock back and forth in my bed to distract myself until help arrived. Somehow the movement helped. One of the nurses answered my call and once I had told him what was wrong, he asked me to score the pain, on a scale of one to ten where ten is the worst pain you have ever experienced. I managed to stammer out, "N-n-n-n-nine-and-a-half." Even at that point I thought I had better keep that extra half back in case it got even worse.

I was given morphine and next morning on ward rounds the attention changed from my throwing up or belting to the toilet to my now completely immobile shoulder. Oh joy. You really do get stunning service as a cancer patient. The duty doctor immediately asked for a physio to come and see me, which they did, but said I would have to be referred as an out-patient once I was home. Not much help there then. In times like this I have always turned to complementary therapies, but that was pretty hard in hospital. I was already feeling that my body had switched itself off, which was pretty frightening – you can only go so long without eating or drinking and I really did want to feel well so I could go home. It was a real Catch 22 situation: I wouldn't be allowed home until I was stronger and putting weight back on, but by staying in hospital I was getting worse not better. The whole process of trying to get myself well in a drug-free fashion became a hallmark of my hospital stay.

Chat Room

Blog #33 7th July, 2013

This is my fifth attempt at a blog in the last two weeks, so please don't think I haven't been trying. Now, finally home, I am summoning together little bits of energy into a useful chunk that might actually allow me to finish. You wouldn't believe how much energy it takes to a) sit upright to type and b) use both hands to type. I have to keep stopping to lean on one hand and continue typing with the other hand. And that is only these few words so far. Only a couple of thousand more to go then!

One of the problems with trying to blog from hospital was that, as my ever-so-carefully-monitored health was changing on a daily, if not hourly basis, anything I found the energy to write became old news immediately. Now from the other side of my twenty-three day stay I can give you a synopsis of the highs (?) and lows of the last two weeks and spare you the minute by minute pain of it all. Maybe I can squeeze all that into the book, which will rapidly be approaching doorstop dimensions if I carry on like this!

Reading back over the blogs I had started to write, but run out of energy to finish, it all seems like such old news; my exuberance at coming through the process so well and apparently unscathed was totally undermined by the high temperature 'spikes' that followed, the best one of all being 40.2 degrees C. I looked that one up as I still work on old money for temperature, and was astounded to see it is about 104 degrees F. No wonder they got a bit excited. My Hickman lines have now come out – yes! – as they were a possible source of infection, but the best thing of all about that is that I no longer feel like one of those budget aliens from the early days of Star Trek, with spurious wires coming out of my skin.

The 23 days split neatly into Days 7 down to Zero, and The Rest, during which anything could, and did, happen. From about Day + 3, I was neutropenic, which apart from making me feel absolutely rubbish also meant I was absolutely definitely confined to quarters. I was starting to get some serious cabin fever after over a week of gazing out over a sweet little lake and tantalising views of the balcony. I don't care if the weather was horrible, I wanted to breathe it and experience it for myself just to know it was so. The far side of the balcony looks out over the lake, and I could see a tiny bit of it from my room. The sun rises directly over the lake and I witnessed some truly spectacular sunrises in my time here. I got Stephen to bring in my yoga mat and I was speaking with great excitement of doing my yoga practice facing the rising sun, on the summer Solstice. That was silly – plans again, see? And they laughed… Come the Great Day I was feeling very far from celebrating anything, especially if it involved moving.

The isolation part is so weird. I was so lucky to have access to the world via my mobile etc. but during isolation I was totally reliant on whatever people are able to take out or bring into the room. The fridge idea was brilliant. Stephen pitched up with smoothies, juices and waters, and quickly added some ready meals, milk and whatever else I happened to fancy. Being able to make my own cafetière coffee made a massive difference as it was one more familiar taste or routine to make me feel at home.

Food was, of course, a battle ground. Well that isn't entirely true – the food was there, it's just that I wasn't prepared to eat it. Stephen brought home cooked food in for me during the first week, then for several days as I hit the low part of the process I couldn't face eating anything; my appetite came back before the temperature spikes hit and I wanted to make up for lost time! Access to the 'Special Menu' was only via The Dietician, who, despite repeated requests from the ward had failed to materialise apparently on the grounds of being 'very busy' and also that I wasn't yet malnourished enough to be worthy of a visit. In the beginning I was interested in talking to her because of the absolute mess that the food and the menu is in – but it had now got to the point where I just wanted a cooked breakfast and she was the only way to get it. More requests from the ward and then finally a look alike from a Vogue catalogue came in and announced she was a student dietician and her mission was to see how the hospital could help me to increase my weight by providing some more varied food. Sweet. She knew all about my thoughts on hospital food. Clearly the feedback form did actually get fed back and they must have figured that the best way to deal with it would be to send in a newbie so that nobody with a fully paid job had to come to discuss things that couldn't be changed anyway.

And it worked really well. There have been many surprises in these last few weeks and this was one of them. Far from being a newbie without a clue, Chrissie was a bright, engaged and engaging student who is obviously headed for far greater career vistas than anything the NHS has to offer. Or at least I do hope so. She completely understood the reasons I eat the way I do at home and what I was hoping to achieve when I got out of there. We had a good chat about no carbs, the 5:2 diet and other areas of interest, and jointly came to the conclusion this stay was more about survival tactics than anything else.

I discovered that the dietician's role in the hospital is to find creative ways with very poor products to tempt underweight patients to put on a bit of weight. Very much along the two scoops of ice cream, extra butter on your toast kind of thing than any chance of improving what is sent up. She didn't have access to anything more exciting on the menu than I already knew about but she swiftly offered to order me bacon and egg for breakfast. After days and days of Readibrek I was so ready for that. Which is just as well, because you have to Ask For It To Be Stopped if you want a break, and that of course implies that you would also have to Ask For It Again if necessary. So the following morning the cooked breakfast materialised, borne aloft by Maitre d'Dot and I did manage to eat a few mouthfuls of it; I was shocked at how much my appetite had shrunk.

By far the weirdest thing about isolation is the way your words are taken out of the room by the people that come into it. From my perspective, I was gently asking little questions like, how do I get access to a reflexologist in here, and can I stick a sign on the door so that I'm not disturbed for a bit, to get some meditation in? Small conversations with nurses about their lives, their hopes and dreams – little bits and pieces that make the world go round, that we don't usually give a lot of attention to. What I was in no way prepared for was the way in which this spread like wildfire out on the nurses' station. My room suddenly became a kind of 'chat room', a safe place for the nurses to retreat to when the going got tough outside. My interest in complementary therapies became big news in a way it hadn't with my shorter stays, and even the doctors were coming in to talk about it.

One of the massive side effects of the Mephalin is that it destroys the gastro-intestinal tract – literally. What you are left with is a gooey, disgusting mess in your mouth which is a million times worse than the worst case of thrush you have ever had. Think Jabba the Hut, all the way down to the exit point. I had been told I could have loads of different mouthwashes and painkillers, even a morphine pump if necessary as I would find it almost impossible to swallow. I rejected the mouthwashes from the outset as they were loaded with saccharine and flavouring and said I would manage with a saline mouthwash. And my secret weapon, Vitamin A drops. These had prevented any mouth issues whatsoever throughout the rest of my chemo and I was hoping they would bring salvation now. And they did in spades. The worst I had was the Jabba the Hut mouth, which was deeply unpleasant, but absolutely nothing like as bad as everyone expected. This in itself created a stir as it has never happened before.

A group of doctors came in one day in a bizarre combination of 'show and tell' and 'I told you so'. I duly exhibited my ulcer and sore-free mouth (again) and the senior one looked really baffled and disbelieving. It is strange to observe a hospital consultant faced with something she doesn't really want to see. Two of them were grinning like Cheshire cats, as they had an idea of what was about to happen, whilst the third was struggling with the very obvious proof that something outside the system had prevented me from suffering from the biggest issue that crops up after stem cell transplant. I was having a stronger day so I decided to tell it like it is. I seized the little bottle of Vitamin A drops off the fridge and waved it under her nose, saying, "I'm not presuming to tell you your job (brave!), but this is all you need to do. You shouldn't be having people going through such pain that they need morphine pumps, when 1 drop of this a day will stop all their problems. Don't do complicated research, you can see it works. Don't even ask them, just do it as part of their daily meds. Easy." Gulp. My partners in crime beamed at each other. One suggested using their slush fund to get some, the other said she was just going to go across to the Nutricentre and buy it anyway. Don't know whether they did or not, but it was a splendid moment.

What became apparent during my stay is that there is a huge gap between what the nursing staff (the jury is still out for the doctors as shown above), want to provide for their patients on a more complementary basis and what is available – and there is a massive discrepancy from area to area and even between hospitals within the same county on that level. My desire for a reflexologist really opened a can of worms on this point. Several of the nurses had trained at Poole Hospital, which is a different Trust with a separate budget. At Poole Oncology unit, reflexology and aromatherapy massage are offered free as a service to patients, supplied by the MacMillan unit, *which is based at Christchurch Hospital, where it is also offered free. But it isn't offered at Bournemouth, which is situated between Christchurch and Poole. and is part of the same Trust as Christchurch. How nuts is that?*

One of the nurses knows the reflexologist so was able to put us in touch with each other, and I paid for her to come and give me a treatment. Which was fabulous, but I shouldn't have had to jump through hoops to sort it out for myself. Several of the nursing staff were sufficiently annoyed by my battle that they are thinking of doing special projects to show how important complementary therapies were in patient recovery. I suggested to them that they use the success stories and experiences of other hospitals that already offer these services rather than attempt to re-invent the wheel and try to prove that the therapies work. That would be a complete waste of time; The Royal Marsden, St. Barts, and countless other hospitals have already done the legwork. This battle appears to be about getting someone with budgetary control committed to this level of care. I would imagine it got lopped off the budget at Bournemouth simply because the person doing the budget wasn't interested. Sorry, Bournemouth hospital, not good enough.

I am immensely heartened by all this. Several of the staff are really committed and have asked me to stay in touch to give a hand with their projects. Their enthusiasm has also enabled me – mentally at least – to fit the final piece in the puzzle between allopathic and alternative medicine. This has previously been a battle between the two in my head, and what this whole six months has shown me is that the two disciplines can work together. I am proof of that, so from now on I consider everything outside of 'science' to be 'complementary' rather than 'alternative'. There doesn't have to be a choice – I didn't have that luxury, and this is about taking the best of both.

So – I did eventually make it outside, and spent some lovely time talking to a couple of other patients on the patio. Unbelievably, my story had also reached them from my little isolation suite, which was almost embarrassing. To think that the nurses had carried my story not only to each other and the doctors, but to other patients, was humbling in the extreme. I think it has given me a pretty good direction to follow in the coming months.

My recovery is going to be exceedingly slow, but I have lots to occupy myself. I am fascinated by the way human beings cope in situations like the one I have just been through. To be violated from the inside out by the drugs and the outside in by the medical processes leaves one feeling totally open, psychically, spiritually and emotionally too. It was in those deepest, darkest and most uncomfortable moments when I was completely alone that I started to wonder how I held it all together. I will have much to meditate upon as I regain my strength.

Be well and enjoy the sun!
Mxx

The days dragged by and eventually the only thing that was keeping me in was my spiking temperature. It was really strange. I would be fine for most of the day and early evening, then during the night it would suddenly rise. This meant that every day I was thinking they would surely let me go home, but come the morning my temperature was stubbornly keeping me in isolation. However – I guess the doctors are used to this. One of them, a lovely registrar in her final year, who is destined for very high places indeed, came in to say that the problem was probably in my Hickman lines and that she was going to take them out that afternoon. I was so excited. It was a very uncomfortable little operation but at least I was free! The lines were sent away to be tested and one of them was found to be the source of the infection. I was already on antibiotics so it was just a question of them starting to work and I could really think about going home.

There was also the problem of my weight of course, and the fact that I couldn't keep anything down when I did manage to eat. I was sure that I just needed to be home, so as the source of the infection had been excised from my body I put 'Operation Going Home' into action. The first thing I stopped was the four-hourly blood pressure checks. My blood pressure had been no cause for concern for most of my stay, and the constant inflating of the cuff was making my arms so sore they started to ache as soon as the process started. So I refused to have it taken. I told the duty doctor that they could take it once a day and no more. He grinned. I think he knew what was coming. The next day he came in and I said I was ready to go home as I was 'failing to thrive' in the hospital environment. He was great, actually. I reminded him that we were very sensible people and that I had a vested interest in being well.

Once you are in the care of the doctors it is so hard to keep hold of any sense of responsibility or, that lovely word, control. I mentioned that in all the time I was having the chemo cycles I hadn't been hospitalised once for any problems between treatments; we also live 20 minutes from the hospital so, if necessary, I could get there quickly in an emergency. He said, "One more day then," and went out smiling. The first thing I did was put Fenella Flamingo away, which gave a very strong message to everybody as she was a very powerful, if silent, part of my support team. I started to take down and put away the various personal effects I had spread around the place, so by the next day it was all looking quite bare. Stephen arrived nice and early, and the nurses, bless their cotton socks, had quietly accumulated all the medicines I would need from the pharmacy so we wouldn't have to wait for them to be brought up on the day. The doctor came in, saw the bare room, grinned, and said I could go. What an amazing feeling. By the time we were really packed up and ready there were quite a few people around outside by the nurses station. There were many hugs and a lot of waving and smiling, and we finally made our way out to the sunshine.

By the time I left the ward the whole issue of complementary therapy had become a really hot topic. It seemed that several of the nurses were planning on doing special projects on therapies as a way of raising awareness in the medical profession. It was interesting that the nursing staff were, on the whole, very open to anything that would help us to recover more quickly – they were genuinely interested, and wanted to be able to offer resources that are available in other hospitals. It is the level above the nursing staff that is the problem. Finance and politics at that level act as the cork in the bottle that stops the genie of complementary medicine escaping. But what is so ridiculous, and this is something I really don't understand, is that treatments available at one hospital are viewed with extreme scepticism at Bournemouth. If the Royal Marsden has discovered that acupuncture or reflexology helps patients with chemo-induced sickness, one would think it would be common practice to offer it on all cancer wards. And its use would actually help finances and budgets, as we wouldn't need the expensive drugs that are currently trawled out at every opportunity. The whole can of worms was much too big for me to take on while I was still having treatment. As I read these blogs back to put them into this book I find the fire is still there to lobby for change; I am still incensed at the old-fashioned attitudes I encountered, but at least it kept me amused and busy. When my strength and stamina have fully returned – I will be ready for the fight!

It was so wonderful to be home. The constant intrusions of life in hospital had left me exhausted at a very deep level. As I have mentioned in numerous places, I really need a lot of peace and silence – the knowledge that I won't be interrupted brings a special kind of peace even when I'm not ill, so it was truly wonderful to relax into that security. Stephen looked after my every need and was always there to hold me when the tears of frustration overflowed. I had lost a lot of weight through not eating, and I was so weak I could hardly walk anywhere without needing to sit down almost immediately. I was distressed at the way my muscles had wasted and was shocked when I saw myself in a full length mirror for the first time. I was as scrawny and hunched over as an old woman, with the lack of energy to match. This was a huge lesson in allowing other people to help and I had to work very hard at it – I find it almost impossible to sit down when others are doing household chores, but my debilitation meant I had no choice. I realised that 'not-doing' is very much harder than 'doing', which distracts the mind wonderfully; constant activity is a very effective way of keeping the world at arm's length. Does that ring any bells?

My early days at home were filled with sleep, mindfulness practice, then as some light relief, a humungous amount of 'chick lit'. Good chick lit is like chicken soup for the soul. I have a permanent reading pile of serious books which is about three feet high, but at this stage the only words my poor, undernourished brain could cope with were those designed to float gently into my mind with the express mission of bringing a smile to my face or laughter to my lips. I know that laughter is a really important part of health – and thus recovery – that's why I don't hold back on the graveyard humour. I emailed several of the authors to say how much I loved reading their books while I was ill, and I had such lovely replies. They were delighted to know they had cheered me up and eased my way. There is plenty of time to read the more serious books and to be honest, there are only so many cancer books one can read in a given period. So life trundled on...

The Long Haul back to Health

Blog #34 24th July, 2013

It has been a l-o-n-g and boring few weeks, marked only by my birthday (thanks for all the good wishes via Facebook etc.) and the tiny little improvements I've noticed on a daily basis. When I first came out of hospital I couldn't walk anywhere around the flat without pausing for a pit stop en route, which drove me mad. After weeks of inactivity in hospital I was desperate for a change of scenery, so there was an element of novelty in being able to wander from one room to another – except by the time I'd got to the kitchen from the lounge (15 feet?) I came over all useless and had to sit at the kitchen table with my head down to recover. A big part of this was weakness from not eating as it is only in the last four of five days that I have really managed to get rid of the nausea. Or it was time for it to leave me, whatever.

I was horrified at what the Mephalin had done to my GI tract. The medics weren't kidding when they said it would be destroyed, but I knew I needed to eat so that my body could expel the toxins and start to heal. Not quite so easily done when I was being sick every day and what food I did manage to get down often didn't even touch the sides before it reappeared. I needed the heavy duty anti-emetics from the hospital at first, but I really wanted to come off those so I also tried two homeopathic remedies, Nux Vom (lovely name) and Arsenicum. Neither of these had much effect so I moved on to Cocculus, which was a real find. Apparently it is really good for seasickness too – talking of which I also tried Lyn's sea sickness wrist bands, as well as massaging the relevant acupressure points on my hands. I'm not sure which helped most really, although I did take the Cocculus with me on my first few outings as I found that the hollow feeling in my stomach is what prompted the nausea. And it was hollow most of the time because I was eating so little, and I was eating so little because I felt sick… It is really hard to keep your spirits up at these times; menu planning when you are busy working full time can be a real chore, but when you lose your taste for food, and the meals which used to help structure each day have morphed into hourly attempts to eat a few mouthfuls, you really crave the normality and routine.

My weight was dropping at the rate of about a pound a day and I had already lost nearly two stone. In one way I was delighted as having two children and enjoying several extremely decadent cruises had increased my weight more than I wanted, but this was going to the other extreme. I knew I had to stabilise my eating and weight in order to start recovering. I tried to make sure I ate something every hour, even if it was only a spoonful of very well-chewed, steamed vegetables. The totally useless and conflicting advice from hospital was to increase dairy – have milky drinks, add butter to vegetables, eat rich cakes. Whoever thought that up was seriously having a laugh because it is the last thing a chemo patient can tolerate. And, even more ridiculous, my consultant said that my insides were like a newborn baby so dairy wouldn't be good. Did you know there is 300% more protein in cow's milk than human milk? Not that I was going that far, but you get the point…that cow's milk is designed for baby cows, not humans. Er – hello?! Someone inform the dieticians and nurses! This lack of support absolutely infuriates me. All the protein drinks in hospital are milk-based, so they make you – after me, 'Sick!'

Anyway, enough of the sickness. I'm sick of thinking about it and you are no doubt sick of hearing about it. Suffice to say that I have clawed my way back to being able to eat more or less normally and have managed to put on three pounds this week which is a huge leap in the right direction. I am enjoying food again and last night we actually went out for a curry – how daring is that? I was also at work for my first full day today, although taking it very easily. And still eating every hour as my body is playing catch up on the calories. I have started to do a few little exercises every day to start building up some stamina and to try and beat my poor saggy muscles into a semblance of their former selves. My body has completely changed shape and I'm delighted to say that I plan on keeping it this way (except for toning up) and will thus have to go shopping for more clothes. Shame :-)

We are also just into our first complete week since January with no hospital visits. My appointment last week went really well so I was allowed off for good behaviour until next Monday. You cannot believe how good that feels. Apparently there could be a bit of a dip in my blood results in weeks six to ten after transplant (so basically August), when the mature cells that were in the transplant mix will have died off and the new stem cells will be called upon to show their mettle, but one of the good things about eat-

201

ing better is that I can take my supplements again. So I am disregarding that particular warning, or at least not giving it due attention, and in the meantime ramping up the nutrition. I am very anxious to get the remaining chemo out of my system, so to that end have been juicing and also taking Active Zeolite, which is supposed to help remove heavy metals and toxins like chemo.

I've also been skin brushing every day and having Epsom Salts baths. Have you tried them? Amazing. I recommend you try the baths. Add a good mugful of Epsom Salts to the water along with a few drops of a nice essential oil – I use Rose Otto as it smells so delicious – but keep the temperature moderate. The salts make you sweat profusely, then when you get out you need to make a dash for the toilet. Just a warning, but it really does work, and my skin is starting to show its appreciation. It is starting to look a lot healthier, but a reaction to the chemo has also left it darker, so I look really tanned. Result! So I look skinny and tanned and all I had to do was spend 23 days in hospital having noxious drugs pumped into me. See? Always a silver lining!

I find I am very weary of all this now though. Both Stephen and I need a break from it, and although I can't fly and have to stay out of the sun and can't tax myself physically and have to be very careful about catching bugs from other people and still have to turn up for appointments, we are squeezing in a little break at the beginning of September, hopefully to the Isle of Wight. We desperately need a change of scenery and freedom from the reminders of the last seven months. Some hair would help the sense of normality, as I am heartily sick of scarves, but I know that is only a matter of time. I really can't imagine what it will feel like to have hair again, but I am looking forward to the sensation. We should be able to get away for longer, and to more exciting climes, at the end of the year. With hair!

I thought I would be spending this period eagerly researching and adding bits to my blog to make it into a book, as promised, but I am finding I have a curious resistance to doing so. I know, to a certain extent, this is part of my very cardinal, 'what's next?' type of personality; I never checked my work at school, because, having completed it I considered the job to be done and I wanted to move on to something a lot more exciting. That definitely cost me a lot of marks. But there is something more going on here. There is a part of me that has no desire to revisit the upset and trauma of the last seven months, even though I know a lot of the story hasn't been told. I was inspired at the time and ready to fight for what I felt I needed because I was so incensed that I couldn't easily get it, or that the knowledge wasn't readily available. I imagine this is all just a reaction, and the afore-mentioned weariness, to what has been going on, and that probably all I need is to continue resting. Chemo also affects the brain, and whilst I haven't been as 'out of it' as some people are, something has definitely taken the edge of my mental, as well as physical stamina. It isn't something one would normally think about, but it does take a lot of energy to process thought, which is probably why it has taken me so long to write this blog!

On that note I will retreat to my semi-convalescence, but I will be in touch more as my brain resurfaces!

Wishing you happiness and health

Margaret

Stretching Myself

Blog #35 4th August, 2013

Lots of highs and lows this week, as anyone with a long term illness or convalescing will appreciate. Good days are almost always followed by bad days simply because, if you are anything like me, you overdo it on the good days, which equals at least one step backwards for the next few days. Grrrr. It is SO hard to pace myself. Imagine being denied sweets, wine, cakes, whatever floats your boat, for absolutely months, nay years, then someone opens the doors to the store room and away you go. I defy any normal person not to overdo it. By about Monday I was just recovering from the curry adventure last week which really, really upset my newly developed GI tract (why is it always a curry night which is my undoing?), which was just as well as we had someone coming to clean the carpets on Wednesday, and of course there is a fair amount of moving around to do in preparation. Several house parties have taken their toll on the carpet and don't even get me started on the chocolate fountain. Don't ever, ever, ever even consider getting one unless you have Dikki bibs and wall to wall plastic sheeting at the ready. And that is just for the adults! Anyway, good result by the end of the day. Lovely sparkly clean carpets.

Making some attempt to pace myself, on Thursday I kind of rested. Earlier in the week I had a phone call from the physio department at the local hospital saying they had a cancellation for Thursday morning – I had completely forgotten that one of the consultants from Ward 11 had referred me for my shoulder (when it was so painful after the stem cell transplant) so I trotted off to Christchurch Hospital for my 9.30 appointment. Nice to have a change of scenery from Bournemouth. I must admit I was in two minds about accepting the appointment as, hand on heart and apologies to all the hard working physios out there, physio has never done much for me. But, as you may have noticed in the previous blogs, I have a new attitude which embraces the best of all options in healthcare. I also like to think I am slightly more charitable and less critical then I used to be, so I decided to go along and see what I could learn.

The problem with my shoulder started waaaay back about 25 years ago when I was really quite fit and before I had the boys. I awoke one morning to excruciating pain in my shoulder, which nobody, in the short term, seemed able to cure. The pain finally receded to something more manageable but I could hardly use my right arm. After several months I went to see a cranial osteopath friend of my brother who was absolutely magnificent and sorted the problem out in a couple of visits. Fast forward a couple of decades, and I am finding that a few years of dancing (especially ballroom, which does put you in the oddest posture), a lot more desk work and possibly not as much yoga as should be practised (!) are leading to more and more episodes of neck and shoulder problems. The long stay in hospital, where I was immobile for several days at a time due to sickness, was really the icing on the cake, so I am back to having limited use of my arm and quite a lot of pain. I love the way I answer my own questions when I write this blog. I was about to say that I haven't visited a cranial osteopath since I moved to Bournemouth (which is the obvious answer to the current problem) because there wasn't anyone I had been drawn to, but then I realised I have in fact discovered someone in the last few weeks. Funny that. ANYWAY, sorry to ramble, but there will eventually be a point to all this. I went to the physio because I thought that knowing about the mechanical side of what had gone wrong might be useful in my attempts to heal the problem myself. BTW I tried the Bowen Technique last week (not enough space here to explain it, so Google it if you are interested), but unusually for me, it didn't have any effect at all. I should go back for more, in all fairness, but I feel more drawn to cranial osteopathy now.

The physio was really helpful and picked out things like the fact that I am getting slightly hunched due to work at the computer. That horrified me. I know that the shoulder problem comes from the vertebra between my shoulder blades, and the exercise he gave me ably demonstrated this because I could feel the stretch up my back. Read the next sentence then find a wall and try it. Stand with your heels, bottom, shoulders (flat) and head against the wall; stretch up from the back of your neck so your chin is very slightly tucked in. Ouch. He gave me lots of other very easy exercises to try to gently start my shoulder moving again. I have another appointment in September, so lots of time to practise. More of this in a moment.

From a strictly girlie point of view the other exciting thing that happened after physio was that I had my first manicure in eight months. I know it seems a trivial thing, but as there is absolutely no point me going to a hairdresser at the moment I needed to find somewhere for a bit of pampering. Also, I was prevented from wearing nail varnish during my treatment because at every visit (and four times a day during stays on the ward), part of the 'obs' that are done involve an oxygen sensor being clipped on a finger – and it doesn't work through nail varnish. I could be wrong here, and I am sure the guys will correct me if so, but I think chemotherapy treatment is more de-humanising for women than it is for men. As a woman, losing my hair has been a massive thing. Yes, I have had fun with the scarves and hats, but I feel curiously vulnerable and very obviously a chemo patient; a bald man isn't necessarily noticeable, whereas a woman – even bedecked in a pretty scarf – especially when her eyebrows have disappeared too, does stand out. (Tried the eyebrow pencil and that really doesn't do it.) Add to that the ban on nail varnish and it takes a lot away from the fun side of being a woman at a time when one's self-esteem is in huge need of propping up. However, I am delighted to report that my eyebrows have already reappeared and my hair is starting to sprout. When it gets to the length where it doesn't scare small children or old people I will try leaving my scarves at home and brave the world, Sinead O'Connor style.

So. Friday dawned and as you can imagine I felt quite tired from the week's exertions and decided to have a nice relaxing day at home. I have been literally itching to do some yoga again and Friday felt like the day to start. As lymphoma is a cancer of the lymphatic system, I had to stop most kinds of exercise during my treatment – the last thing I wanted was to stimulate a system which could circulate cancerous cells around my body. I'm neither the fittest nor the most athletic person on the planet, but the lack of activity over such a long time was driving me crazy. As I am now unofficially in remission (to be confirmed by the PET scan in a few months), I have tried a few teeny stretches recently but even those took a lot of effort in my currently weakened state, so I knew I had to be careful. The sun was shining so I opened the conservatory doors to let in the warm breeze, laid my yoga mat to face the sun, and started a new meditation CD I have been wanting to try. I know from previous experience that unresolved emotions are held within the body and that once you start to free up the knots and blocks within, they will start to surface. I wanted to give them ample opportunity to do so. I decided to stick to very simple stretches, interspersed with long periods of relaxation laying Alexander Technique-fashion at the end of each one, and include the new stretches I had learnt from the physio where appropriate. I am glad I set my sights so low :-(.

Having previously been able to fold myself in half at the drop of a hat, I was horrified that while sitting with my legs out in front of me I could barely reach my ankles, let alone get my head to my knees. No chance! The CD I had chosen was perfect: 'Earth' by Alex Theory, part of his Full Spectrum Sound Healing series. The slow drumbeat encouraged me to calm my thoughts and allow my body to sink into the floor. Having done many years of yoga with Swamiji I can still hear her voice even now when I practise, and it is such a help. I focused on allowing my body to relax down into the postures; I could feel the muscles creaking as they were finally given the space and time to unfurl, and oh my goodness did the emotions pour forth.

My poor, poor body. I didn't realise it had gone so badly and totally into shutdown as a means of self-defence. Way back when I first had the problem with my shoulder, the cranial osteopath said it was the culmination of a lot of issues that had gone unresolved – the straw that broke the camel's back. It struck me as I relaxed into the posture that it had served its purpose and given me the same message again. As I breathed into my back, encouraging the muscles to open and relax it felt as though a part of me was peering out, like a child hiding behind a curtain: "Is it safe to come out now?" Yes, it was safe. Within seconds the tears were flowing. I think they were tears of relief as it felt really good and didn't turn into the helpless sobbing of fear and desperation. Been there, done that. I wanted to stay in that position and just let it happen, so I did, dripping tears all over the knees I couldn't reach. I realised that through all these months when you lovely people having been saying nice things like how brave and inspirational I am, I have in reality just been coping in the only way I can. Shutdown. At all costs keep going and deal with the fallout later. Well the time to face the fallout has arrived, and I must say I am glad. I have the time, the resources, and a lovely clean carpet on which to relax to my heart's content.
Thank you for your company on this incredible journey.
With love
Margaret xx

Well – in between the teardrops exploding and some serious pampering I also found a bit of time to reach out to others. Judy had recently had a cataract operation and it felt really good to give her some support. She was unable to drive so for a couple of weekends we managed to raid Waitrose and deliver some groceries to her; she lives out in the middle of nowhere and it was lovely to drive out into the countryside. And it felt so good doing something for somebody else. My world had shrunk beyond belief and I was still finding it a bit intimidating being out amongst the natives and felt extremely worried about the slightest cough or sneeze. I was eager to push out my boundaries again as I had no more chemo to get fit for – I was out of treatment and it felt wonderful. Scary but wonderful. Of course that meant I pushed the boundaries a bit too far too quickly.

Four Steps Back

Blog #36 18th August, 2013

Honestly. Will I never learn? What comes before running? Walking. What comes before curries and chillies? Nice bland food. Whoops, I did it again. You may remember that I recently had a bad few days after our first night out in many months, to a curry restaurant. I recovered from that, and following my very successful visit to my newly found cranial osteopath, by last Tuesday I was feeling on top of the world and almost like my old self. Then the stupidest suggestion in the whole world came out – I fancied a homemade Mexican beef chilli. Not very spicy, just a nice, beefy change from the endless round of vegetables, fish and chicken. And a glass of wine. Yep – that's how nearly back to normal I was feeling, and I must confess, desperately fed up of being a convalescent. It didn't take many hours for my poor system to start objecting, and now, a week later, I am still repairing the damage and I must confess I haven't got very far. It feels just like when you get a really bad stomach bug – like you've been kicked in the stomach – which isn't the slightest bit conducive to eating, so my weight is dropping again, and I am back to eating teeny portions every hour or so.

The obvious answer to all of this is that my patience is being tested, and because I don't appear to have learnt the lesson yet it is being repeated until I do so. As someone who was at the back of the queue when patience was handed out it is unbelievably difficult for me to rein in my enthusiasm once I start to feel better. Isn't everyone like that? Surely it isn't just me. I start to feel better = I do more = I feel even better = I do more... In my mind that is how it is supposed to go, and being constantly forced to focus on the present and having even very small goals that are still unreachable is driving me crazy. Making arrangements to see friends always has to be tempered with the proviso that we have to see how I am on the day. I can't be doing with this. But the only way through it is to be good and give my insides a chance to heal. As someone at the hospital put it, "If you wouldn't feed it to a baby you were weaning, don't eat it." Fabulous.

I had my second appointment with the cranial osteopath on Monday, during which we got talking about the practice of Mindfulness. I am find-

ing Mindfulness very helpful in coping with the future, as in when you are trying not to worry about it in advance. It is easy then to take each moment for what it is, one moment at a time. Somehow the discipline of not worrying is very comforting. But what about when you do want to think about the future? To dream, to plot and scheme, to plan? I obviously haven't come to the right bit in the teachings yet which shows you how to do this. Any guidance from Buddhist readers would be most helpful here, as I suspect I am getting into deep water.

At the first diagnosis, cancer robs you of the future you had assumed was yours. You are forced to think in terms of one day at a time, one treatment at a time, because it is too painful to think about the future with conviction. At least I found it so. I didn't have the strength to assume I would be in that future when I was in so much shock, as it meant I had to think about my loved ones and how they would cope if I don't make it through all this. Now I am finding my old dreams and aspirations coming back, which is lovely, but of course they have a slightly different tag attached. None of us know what the future holds, but a cancer patient knows it even less, if that is possible. How do I dream of the future, and all the things I would love to be in it without also dragging in the consequences of the last eight months and their associated concerns? Can I dream of the future selectively? That would be fun – leave out all the potentially bad bits. I guess that is what day dreaming is. Be aware that I have a lot of time on my hands just now; I can't really go into work with my innards in this fragile state so my mind is working overtime and galloping way ahead of my body. This is where writing the blog is so useful. Having got to this point it is blazingly obvious to me that what I should be doing is some very gentle yoga and meditation to bring my mind under control and to ease my body. I would never have got there just sitting and thinking about it on my own, so thank you for keeping me company though the rambling.

As I am cautiously starting to feel a tiny bit better I have managed to think about turning the blog into a book, and I am really pleased to say that I have now managed to write the first Chapter. It was an incredibly emotional experience as I trawled through the period from New Orleans up to the diagnosis in December, and it occurred to me how attached we are to finding the cause of our illnesses. Think about the last time you had a cold or tummy bug; I bet the first thing you did was try to remember all the people you had been in contact with who might have been ill. It is no different with cancer, which I know is crazy, but it is true. Given that by 2020 apparently 1 in 2 of us will have succumbed to it in one form or another (it is currently 1 in 3) it is not beyond the realms of reason that we should do all we can to protect ourselves against either getting it, or a relapse if we have already had it.

We all have the potential within us to develop cancer, and it takes a specific set of circumstances for a cell to turn cancerous – and apart from obvious disasters like Fukushima, those circumstances will be unique to each individual. If we could know with any certainty what those are it would save an awful lot of lives. In my particular case I am still totally fixated on having become ill in New Orleans, and I only realised how firmly attached I still am to that idea when I was writing the Prologue. There is a part of me that thinks it is something I should really be getting over, but there are some things of note that do relate specifically to that location. I apologise in advance to anyone who loves New Orleans, but it is an incredibly toxic place. Yes, the music, arts and general creativity is fabulous, but for me the French Quarter, which is the only part I have seen, has a horribly murky and troublesome past and I can't help feeling that the physical upheaval and flooding caused by Hurricane Katrina has brought a lot of that energy to the surface. I was beginning to think that I was alone in feeling like this about a city that most other people seem to love. At least – it didn't affect them as badly as it did me. Then Stephen brought home a book by Jennie Sherwin called Intentional Healing: One Woman's Path to Higher Consciousness and Freedom from Environmental and Other Chronic illnesses. Jennie was a woman who was becoming sicker and sicker from undiagnosable health issues to the point where she could barely function. It is a complicated (and fascinating) picture which is built up in many layers, but Jennie was able to pinpoint a particular trigger and this is where I really sat up and took notice. Her story begins when her husband's job took them to New Orleans. Their home was to be given a standard treatment of pesticides, something which is required on a regular basis in all public buildings as well as private dwellings, because of the climate. Already beginning to show signs of several allergies, Jennie was quite rightly concerned about the effect these could have but was reassured that the chemicals are quite safe around humans. How often have we heard that one?

As Jennie's story progresses we discover that her illness is, in fact, directly related to the type II pyrethroids that were used in her home. Pyre-

throids are known to be carcinogenic. Mantle Cell Lymphoma is now known to be caused by exposure to pesticides and herbicides. Where does all this get me? No idea. Clearly – well at least as far as I am aware – nobody else developed cancer after the conference, so presumably my immune system was already debilitated when I got there. Which is highly possible as I wasn't feeling fantastic when we left home. So maybe New Orleans was my own unique trigger. In the light of Jennie's book, it is looking very much like it could be, so in some very small way, rightly or wrongly, I feel exonerated for blaming New Orleans as the source of my illness.

So while I need to concentrate on getting my body as strong as possible and building my immune system up, I also need to make sure that I really do detox thoroughly. I have my regular appointment with the wonderful Joe tomorrow so I will ask him what he thinks. I will report back!
Wishing you good health
Margaret xx

Well, somewhat predictably, Joe wanted me to get fitter and stronger, and especially for my skin to be back to normal before I went off to any fancy detox regimes. But he wasn't against the idea, which is heartening. I did see the sense in his point of view – this slowing down to allow myself to heal was such an alien concept and I was still trying to belt around as if I was well. The reality of my fragility became obvious as August progressed. A treatment as savage as high dose chemotherapy – especially on an already debilitated body – causes immense damage at every level. It really messed with my head that I was being given all these horrendous drugs that in the process of ridding me of the cancer were making me so very ill. It emphasised yet again to me that the battle with cancer is mostly a mental one that demands immense strength and presence of mind. I had been feeling very sick again – almost regressing back to the bad old days after the transplant, only this time the sickness was accompanied by stomach ache. I was taking Omeprazole to help reduce the irritation in my stomach so it would accept food, and one day I had the really bright idea of checking the side effects. The first one was stomach ache. I say again, "What are these people thinking?" I stopped the Omeprazole and the stomach aches disappeared. Allelujah. I cuddled the green calcite Judy had given me back and took Cocculus for the empty sicky feelings, and I very slowly started to make progress.

After reading this post, Bob Makransky sent me a quote from Carlos Castenada's *The Wheel of Time*, in which the terminally ill actor, Julian, is taken into the mountains by the nagual Elias. A nagual in Mesoamerican folk religion is a powerful magician who is able to shapeshift into various animal forms. Elias told Julian that, whilst he couldn't promise to cure him, he could help to extend his life. Julian turned into a vigilant student who was forever treading the narrow path between the more sensual and decadent side of his nature and the instinct to survive. And survive he did, becoming a nagual himself and living to about a hundred and seven years old. Elias says:

> *His fight was not sporadic; it was a most sustained, disciplined struggle to remain balanced. Walking on the edge of the abyss meant the battle of a warrior enhanced to such a degree that every second counted. One single moment of weakness would have thrown the nagual Julian into that abyss.*

Without wishing to seem over-dramatic, that is how it felt to me as I clawed my way back to health.

Hair We Go Again

Blog #37 31st August, 2013

It has been a strange week, but by far the most exciting bit of it has been the realisation that I really do have hair now. In fact this morning I thought, "I really should wash my hair", which after seven months is a very strange concept, I can tell you! I am so pleased to ditch the headscarves. As the warm weather has continued (for which I am deeply grateful, of course) they have become more and more uncomfortable, and somewhat out of place with summer dresses and the like.

It is usually about this time of year I start getting really sad that the summer is ending – mainly because it hasn't even got properly started and I feel I am being grossly short-changed on my sunshine quota. I seem to suffer from SAD so we try to escape for some winter sunshine towards the end of the year – a nice, sunny holiday seems to set me up to last right through until the Spring. This year, however, my wildest dreams have come true, in a funny kind of way. Enforced rest is irritating at the best of times for someone who is usually very active, and it is especially unpleasant when accompanied by an outlook of grey skies and rain. But the British summer of 2013 has excelled itself, so although I am banned from actually sitting in the sun, I have been able to sit outside under the parasol and also enjoy our lovely sunny conservatory. It makes a massive difference to my state of mind, which is still quite fragile.

Enough of the weather, and I promise I won't spend an entire paragraph on it again! I mentioned in the last blog that the exercise of Mindfulness is on the whole, very helpful. However, it is a full time job, and I can't at any point let my guard down – this has to be a life's work. The reason I say this is that it is easy to praise any spiritual exercise when the going is easy. How about when the going gets tough? That's when I get to see how much attention I have been paying in class. My cranial osteopath pointed out that I often use the word 'your' as opposed to 'mine' so I am trying hard to be present in what I write and not fob it off on you. He has a point. Using 'your' is distancing myself and almost conveniently convincing myself I am writing about all of us. This isn't the case, and it is a salutary reminder about coming home to my mind and body. I am leading a reasonably sheltered life at the moment in an attempt to build my weight and strength back up after the last few weeks. Stephen is still doing most of the shopping and I haven't been into work much; what this means is that when I do venture out I feel unexpectedly vulnerable, and suddenly feel swamped by everything and need to cry for no obvious reason at all. Stephen was completely bemused when I accompanied him to Sainsburys last week and returned in tears from an innocuous trip to track down coleslaw. Simple activities like mixing with everyone else in a shop can completely overwhelm me in minutes, as I'm just not used to the amount of energy that is generated by a lot of people rushing around doing their shopping – it underlines just how depleted I still am. I feel the desperate urge to retreat to my safe little bubble at home as soon as possible. This is clearly one of the areas that needs to be worked on, but it is giving me a massive insight into other mental states that I haven't experienced before.

The other thing that cuts straight through my newly acquired mindfulness strategy is the unexpected reminder – when I'm not expecting it – that cancer is out there, alive and extremely strong. We had some really sad news yesterday. A neighbour's daughter was diagnosed with breast cancer a couple of weeks after my own diagnosis – so literally just before Christmas. She had a double mastectomy then chemotherapy for other, multiple tumours, which didn't work. She died two weeks ago. I never even met the lady but I cried for her bravery, and for her family, and railed against the savagery that is cancer. I am part of a support group on Facebook and a few days before this news I had read an equally upsetting post from a member. As far as she was concerned her PET scan results were expected to be fine when she got them the next day; she was so excited about the freedom that knowledge would bring and she was looking forward to a new life, cancer free. The appointment came, and not only was her cancer back, it was so widespread she has been given three months to live. I was appalled. I could still see the two posts, before and after, on my screen. This killer is so insidious. Its first appearance isn't even obvious to most people, and it's like walking around with a ticking bomb inside. I will be having my own PET scan in the next month or so, and whilst we will obviously be delighted if it shows I really am in remission, I can't take that as a guarantee. All it means is that at the point when I was scanned I was clear. I have seen and heard too many stories on the cancer ward to take anything for granted. Please don't think I am being negative. I'm not. I am being realistic about the terror that cancer buries deep in your mind – and it is a terror that I believe can never be expunged.

A fellow astrologer acquainted me with a wonderful phrase many moons ago, and it is perfect for this scenario: This is clearly an AFOG (Another ******* Opportunity for Growth). Yep. A situation I cannot change and have absolutely no choice about, so as somebody famous once said, and I believe I might have said it before, "The only way round this is through it". Harsh but true. Getting through any illness takes at least as much mental strength as it does physical. A possible way that cancer differs from many other illnesses is that one has to be in it for the long term, so it is essential to build up the stamina to keep going – which is about where I am at.

When all this started you will remember I had bags of energy to go out and find alternative remedies and follow up every possible lead that would help me on my way to health. I am absolutely sure that the remedies, the juicing, the change of diet, etc., are what got me through the cycles of chemotherapy in such good shape. I arrived at the stem cell transplant thinking I could get through it in a similar style: a bit of sickness, a bit of feeling grotty. I took their warnings with a massive pinch of salt and expected to be back in action very quickly. Because of this, I was in no way prepared for the long and uphill slog that this last section has become; it must be a bit like getting to the end of a marathon with only a massive hill between you and the finishing line.

The trouble is that I have gone off a lot of the things that worked for me earlier in the treatment. This last month has been especially difficult as I have had to go back to tiny meals every hour or so, although thankfully that is now improving, but my taste buds are still very finicky. I can't face the juices we were making, and I certainly can't stomach the vast platefuls of greenery I was tucking into, so it has been a matter of trying to find what I can tolerate. I lost weight again in recent weeks, which was annoying, especially as I obviously need to be absorbing nutrients from my food to get stronger. I haven't been able to eat enough calories in recent weeks to stop the weight loss, then I remembered the wonders of whey protein. Several people had suggested getting some of the protein drinks we were offered in hospital, but they are all milk based and filled with stuff I really don't want to put into my system – so I dusted off the smoothie maker and we have been having lots of fun with berries, coconut water, soya milk and bananas – and big spoonsful of protein powder. It seems to be starting to work as although I haven't gained any weight, at least I have stopped losing it, and my strength is improving.

The advice from the hospital is to do a tiny bit of exercise each day and gradually increase the amount. I remember the transplant co-ordinator saying that I really wouldn't feel like it but that I needed to push myself. She is so right! I have to say that although I enjoy a certain amount of physical activity when I am well, I would never have made a world class athlete – as soon as it starts to hurt, I stop. I really have no interest in working through the pain barrier or pushing myself that bit further. In fact, I would go so far as to say that I can see the pain threshold approaching and take devious measures to avoid it, like stopping to retie my shoelace. I have many such excuses. But I'm now in an interesting scenario, where again I have to dig deep and change old habits: if I want to get well, I have to push myself – it is the only way to build up stamina, and a few half-hearted leg raises aren't going to do it.

Stephen and I are off on a little jolly next week to the Isle of Wight. He hasn't been before and I last went more years ago than I care to remember, so we are really looking forward to our first adventure since this whole debacle began. We desperately need a change of scenery as we have both spent far too much time within these four walls in recent months. We are staying in a hotel overlooking the beach and will have a sea view and balcony, upon which I am planning to relax with a good book while Stephen goes for some bracing walks. I don't think the hotel has a lift so I am pleased to say that I will have to exert myself on a reasonably regular basis just to get back to the room. All this is good, of course, and I look forward to returning to the blog a bit fitter than when I left J

Wishing you a lovely weekend

Margaret

And so we finally got away. My eating still wasn't very reliable, and this trip would go some way to proving to me that I could function outside of our flat; at home I was still eating every hour or so, and if I didn't eat as soon as I felt a bit hungry I very quickly felt sick. It all seemed a bit precarious to me, and I wasn't sure how I would manage. The first thing I did, of course, was cry when we got there (this seems to be my default setting, but Stephen is very used to it by now). I cried at the relief of actually getting away, and I cried at the way my life had been reduced to this; then I crawled back up from the pit I had just fallen into and started to appreciate both the lovely hotel and the Island.

Travelblog

Listen; there's a hell of a good universe next door: let's go.

Rumi

I thought you might appreciate a bit of a travel blog as a change from the continual angst of a cancer blog :-). My coping strategy of storing wry observations for future use seems to have followed me to the beautiful and sun-kissed Isle of Wight and translated itself into the urge to tell you all about this place.

We dithered for ages over whether to book a holiday or not. The six to ten week 'low' certainly hit me like a sledge hammer, and we didn't dare think of committing to this little break until I was keeping food in and down with a reasonable amount of certainty, and could make it from the lounge to the kitchen without a sit down. And even then we checked that we could cancel with no fee. That is what life is like just now. No guarantees. The main thing to understand about the Isle of Wight (for anyone who is unaware of it) is that it is very old fashioned – much like Cornwall of thirty years ago. The North of the Island is very sailing and yachtie-biased, leaving the very beautiful sub-tropical South for those of us who prefer a less active and less frenetic pace of life. The High Streets are busy and thriving with proper, old-fashioned shops that look as though they have been there for generations. We have driven all the way around the island now, and I am happy to report we have only seen one national chain outlet so far, although I imagine there are others lurking off the main roads. It is a very refreshing change.

Although we live quite close to the sea ourselves, we wanted a hotel which was practically falling into it – which is how we ended up choosing The Wellington Hotel in Ventnor. That and the fact that they included the ferry travel from Lymington in the price of the room. The five mile stretch of water between the mainland and the Isle of Wight is purportedly the most expensive in the world – you are lucky to get a return ticket for a car and passengers for under about £60 (assuming you don't want the 5.am sailing!). Of course we trawled Trip Advisor etc. for reviews of the hotel before we booked it, and we came up with some real anomalies: some people absolutely loved it and the very odd few loathed it and absolutely savaged it online. I do feel sorry for the hard working folk who keep the hospitality industry alive. More of that in a moment. We decided we would take the risk as the hotel looked so lovely – an old Victorian building literally clinging to the hillside above the beach, with every room promising a sea view and most with balconies. As this was our first break of any kind in ages we booked the super deluxe room. Hang the expense!

It was with some trepidation that we pulled up to the hotel and checked in. We were led to our room. Which is gorgeous. The hotel is gorgeous. The views are gorgeous. The staff are gorgeous. OK – yes, the carpets are a bit tatty and old looking on the stairs, and the railings which separate the balconies are a bit rusty. Of course the railings are rusty. The hotel faces the sea and is constantly lashed by fierce winds that decimate paintwork in a matter of months. Don't those detractors realize this? And in the grand scale of things, how important is it? As our most recent holidays have been on fairly swanky cruise ships I was more worried about crunchy white sheets and snowy white towels (which I have grown to love with a passion bordering on obsession), and a clean bathroom (Virgo Moon in action I'm afraid), and on those fronts our room was more than satisfactory. I am sure that some folk are more interested in picking fault than getting on and enjoying their holiday. Or maybe that is their idea of fun. And to be honest, this is a three star hotel. It isn't pretending to be five star or something it isn't, so whilst you might find perfection around every corner in a boutique, mega-expensive hotel, you're probably not going to find it here. I read a cruise review once where the writer said they were pleased to report that their cabin passed 'the white glove test'. Yes. That really does mean that this extremely picky and critical person put on a white glove specifically to check whether the steward had cleaned all those difficult nooks and crannies in their cabin. Complaining about obvious grime is one thing – but imagine checking that you have packed your white gloves! I think that is downright nasty.

I would personally hate to be in the hospitality business. The staff here are gracious and kind and will do anything to help, but they must have to deal with some difficult situations.

For instance, we booked a room with a balcony because we wanted to fall asleep and wake up to the sound of the sea, and to sit outside and enjoy the fresh air during the day when I needed to rest. The couple in the room next door booked a balcony room because they wanted to smoke. The two requirements are mutually exclusive, and the first we knew of it was when our room filled with smoke at 6.00 am on our first morning. We were pretty grumpy, as you can imagine, but didn't especially want to confront our neighbours at that time. And they were probably quite within their rights to smoke – it was probably hotel policy but we hadn't bothered to check. We had a really busy day yesterday and it was only today that we talked about it together; I guess we could have asked for a room change, but we like this room, and why should we be the ones to suffer all the upheaval? But then could we have insisted they move? With a Libra Ascendant this kind of situation is a complete nightmare for me. And I'll never know how it could have worked out as we are leaving tomorrow and didn't bother to ask Reception what they could do about it. I supposed hotel staff get to see and deal with just about everything and they probably wouldn't have batted an eyelid at our dilemma.

We have already decided we want to come back here again. There is loads more to see, as our itinerary has been necessarily limited by my lack of stamina and need for a daily rest. The island seems to be a bit of a mecca for masochistic cyclists (we are talking some very seriously steep hills here, folks), but there is also a coastal path and endless public bridleways to explore. However, lest you think I have been lazing around doing nothing, I would like to say that the private path from the hotel down to the esplanade is made up of 81 steps, which I have personally counted several times. I was told to be very gentle in my attempts to improve my stamina, but there isn't a lot you can do, stranded halfway up a flight of steps. Except sit down for a breather, which is what I did. I have done lots and lots of sitting down since we arrived, but it has been interspersed with quite a bit of walking, much of it uphill. I have to say that the public areas around here are very sensitively designed. It is really easy to find a seat and pretend to be taking in the astounding view whilst calming one's pounding heart – nobody need ever know the truth. We have also found a really nice Tapas Bar, which happens to be at the bottom of the 81 steps. I think I am getting a bit stronger with each climb. Now there's an incentive!

We have both been able to escape the shadow of the last eight months – at least to a certain extent. We have slept well, eaten well, and really enjoyed

being away from old triggers and reminders. Except for one incident yester-
day, but it was kind of okay. We went to Quarr Abbey, a Benedictine mon-
astery on the north of the island. After a fabulous lecture from the guide we
repaired to the onsite tea garden (not fabulous at all), and ended up sharing
a table with two lovely ladies from Texas. One of them has family here and
is a regular visitor, so we talked along those lines for a while, but eventu-
ally the conversation got around to our reason for being here and the whole
cancer story came out. I realized this was the first time I had told anybody
the whole thing, face to face, in the cold light of day. I am always better one
step removed – either writing or talking on the phone – and I found the ex-
perience incredibly difficult. It was so hard not to cry at the more emotional
and difficult points, and I really didn't want to lose it in a public place with
complete strangers. Their sensitive questions and a certain amount of shar-
ing of experiences did make it easier, but again I realized how protected,
and thus vulnerable I have become. It was a good experience though, and
very thought provoking. To be honest, in these weird days post-transplant
and pre-proper hairstyle, going to buy a paper can be a thought-provoking
experience.

Tomorrow we head home, and we are really sad. It has been like going to
a Mediterranean town – blue sea, golden sands, and endless sunshine. We
have been so lucky. And we will be back!
Wishing you sunshine in your heart
Margaret

In Limbo

Before I get side-tracked, I want to draw your attention to the lovely Heather von St James. Heather contacted me via the blog, and asked whether I would help promote Mesothalioma Awareness Day on 26th September by including her link in the blog. This is a particularly rare and lethal form of cancer which has a life expectancy of about 10 months – Heather was diagnosed when her daughter was three and a half months old, and that was seven years ago. Heather is living proof of the importance of a positive and sunny outlook in fighting cancer; she was accused of wearing rose-tinted spectacles and she agreed, saying she had no intention of changing. How lovely. Please do watch her video on her blog at mesothalioma.com/heather then share through social media if you are able.

It was nice to get the boost of her positive energy in my current state of limbo. I went to see Joe on Monday and he was delighted with my blood results but underlined how debilitated my immune system is and how I am really still a bit of a newborn in stem cell transplant terms. I have to say I have come on in leaps and bounds since the Isle of Wight trip, but my new-found energy and hearty appetite tend to lead me astray in terms of thinking I am back to normal now. I might be feeling good, but my system is still busily building new cells and renewing my major organs. Which, frankly, seems rather strange. Periodically I wander off into a philosophical landscape where I wonder how much of the essence of the 'old' me is contained in my new body. Why have some bits of it got lost or destroyed? This troubles me greatly. According to my Bowen therapist my cells have forgotten the Bowen treatments I have had through the years, as my body reacted like a new patient when I started treatment again a few weeks ago. I used to be hypoglycemic and had to watch my sugar intake very carefully – that doesn't seem to be a problem now. Apparently all my childhood vaccines and immunity have been killed off by the pre-transplant chemo, so I will have to have them all again. But how come I still feel and act like 'me'? Surely when the old cells die off naturally in a healthy person, as they do on a cyclical basis, the cells that replace them are somehow programmed to continue the legacy – all that has happened with me is that there was mass genocide and all the stem cells were replaced in one fell swoop. And since all those cells came from me in the first place they must all retain the memories they would have had if they had been replaced at a more normal rate. And if that is the case, why are some things 'remembered' and not others – like the vaccines? Confused? I sure as hell am, and if there is some bright spark out there who isn't and can explain it all to me, please get in touch!

One thing my lovely consultant has done is to book me a PET scan as he wants official confirmation that the cancer has gone. Oh yes. This is the radioactive injection scenario from blog #2, only this time the whole procedure is likely to be a lot more sedate. The appointment is for next Wednesday and is at my usual hospital in Bournemouth. The PET scan roadshow rolls into town every other Wednesday and looks like that decontamination vehicle from the ET film. It comprises several vans connected by covered metal walkways; the walkways lead from the main reception area to separate, somewhat grandly named 'cubicles', where we wait in isolation for the injection to take effect. I have only seen half the process in the vans, as last time the scanner developed a fault and three of us had to belt over to Portsmouth which has a whole wing of the hospital devoted to 'Nuclear Medicine'. So there is much excitement to come; I'm assuming that one of the walkways leads to the scanner, where I'll be given instructions through some squeaky speaker, as nobody wants any contact once the radioactive injection has taken effect. It is a really strange feeling, knowing that I am dangerously radioactive to other people but feeling fine in myself. The worst part of the whole procedure is not being able to eat for six hours before the appointment. I have just started to enjoy food again, but need to eat at regular intervals to avoid feeling queasy. Just like the rest of cancer treatment, this will be a question of mind over matter.

Joe described these early days after transplant as being 'in limbo', and he is absolutely right. After seven months of being in and out of hospital in one way or another, for at least two or three days a week, I have felt almost cast adrift in the last two months. I have gone from being extremely ill to (hopefully) in remission and for that I am eternally grateful, in spite of the barbaric and disgusting drugs. Once we get the scan results I will at least be able to move forward into the next camp and start to get some kind of a life back. At least a part of that life includes getting fit again, and in that department I will be greatly helped by a free 12-week membership to the local sports centre, courtesy of the hospital. I still have a big problem with my frozen right shoulder, which started during the transplant period in hospital and, although it is slowly improving, will prevent me from doing any of the things I really want to in order to get fit: pilates, yoga and swimming are all pretty difficult with one arm :-). I am having physio and Bowen therapy so I am hopeful that recovery is on the horizon. I loved having cranial osteopathy as it was uncovering an awful lot of old patterns and blocks, but unfortunately it is expensive and thus not a long term prospect for a chronic problem like my shoulder.

Just to catch you up on other therapies I have mentioned, remember the Hyperbaric Oxygen Therapy? I was planning on going back to that once my conventional treatment was over, but I had a letter a few weeks back informing me that the local centre has had to close due to funding problems. I'm really sad about that as I was looking forward to renewing my acquaintance with a whole bunch of positive people. Quite apart from the completely bizarre – and cold! – experience of the 'dive' it was enriching to hear their stories and how they cope with a lifelong illness like MS. Sure as hell makes a nice break from cancer! The closest centre is now Portsmouth, which is at least an hour's journey from here, so I will have to give it some thought.

I mentioned my grand plans for all this detox to Joe, who wants me to wait until my skin is back to normal before I go off doing something like that. Personally, I cannot wait to have a swim and sauna, but my skin is being especially troublesome at the moment in spite of my attempts to avoid the sun in recent months. Some of it is quite rough, and all of it is very dry, even though I use a whole load of potions on it, including coconut oil, and bathe and shower in the totally gorgeous but 'friendly' products I was given for my birthday. I also brush my skin every day. Mostly. I guess all this, the shoulder, the skin, the residual tiredness, is just to remind me I am not nearly there yet, and all good things come to those who wait. That was one of my dear mum's favourite expressions, and I bet, when she has time to look in on me from wherever she is now, she is laughing her socks off. I can imagine the purists amongst you itching to comment that of course there won't be socks in the afterlife, but I am betting there are. I gather that heaven/the hereafter/the interlife, whatever you want to call it, is supposed to be nicer and more fun than here, and I really would expect that 'existence' to include

laughter. What would life (or not-life-but-something-else) be without a really good laugh, the sort that makes your tummy ache? You can't be too precious about these things.
Wishing you sunshine and much laughter
Margaret

My confusion over which 'memories' were retained in my body and which were not prompted much discussion over email and on the blog. Bob Makransky had this to say:

As I understand it, memories are not stored in the body but in the Akashic Records – the brain accesses this information in a manner analogous to cloud computing: the information is not stored in the individual computer (body/brain) but on the internet (Akashic Records) – the individual computer (brain) merely accesses this information and acts on it.

It's a shadows on Plato's cave kind of thing. The body and physical brain are like the scoreboard at an athletic event: the scoreboard reflects what's happening on the field, but it doesn't create it – it merely records it. So too our bodies and brains aren't creating anything (all 'creation' takes place in/is directed in dreamless sleep). Our bodies – whether in waking consciousness or dreaming – are merely counters, dummies as it were, walking through a pre-scripted movie which we are projecting from a position in dreamless sleep.

Which somewhat begs the question about me deciding at some inter-life point, where the Akashic Records can be accessed, that I wanted to experience cancer. The Akashic Record, or Book of Life is a dimension of consciousness which contains a record of all the lives the soul has experienced. And out of those experiences comes the desire to reincarnate with perhaps a specific purpose in mind; one which will accelerate soul growth, and which, to be honest, is probably not going to be very pleasant. The Records are accessible through specific exercises and meditations that I have had the privilege to experience with Judy Hall in the past, before I became ill. At that stage I was looking at other blocks and ties I was trying to clear. When I have the strength I would like to go back and examine the reason for experiencing the cancer.

The brilliant thing about working in the Mind, Body, Spirit world is that it is very easy to have these conversations with people – ideas that many outside of it would find difficult to take on board. For the astrologers amongst you, I know that having a Moon/Pluto conjunction in Virgo (which I may just have mentioned once or twice!), drives my thoughts ever deeper. Virgo is a very analytical sign, and in Vedic astrology the Moon rules the mind. So it follows that I need to analyse what is going on at its deepest level. I have never been able to shrug off experiences as 'just life', and move on. You can imagine that this takes me into some pretty dark nights of the soul, even without the experience of dealing with cancer. Fortunately, when these times become particularly intolerable I can reach out to Swamiji. She will always talk some sense to me.

Cheery Thoughts

Blog #40 8th October, 2013

None of us are going to get out of here alive

Swami Ambikananda

I phoned Swamiji the other day for a cheery chat. I am lying. I had spent several more days than I would have liked exploring the doldrums, and I needed somebody to jolt me out of it. One of the things I truly love about Swamiji is that she doesn't hold back. At the hardest times of my life she has been there to say the things nobody else can – the very sentence or sentiment I didn't want to hear, but probably needed to. So I guess I call her for some tough love. It always works.

The particular nugget given above was her response to me saying I'm not coping well with all the uncertainty in my life – and moaning yet again that it feels even more uncertain now because it has been touched, well, stamped all over to be honest, by cancer. I needed guidance for my meditation and an idea of where to focus my thoughts, because, as I discussed in my last post, I feel very much in limbo. I have said many times that I am a control freak, and although its iron grip has been prised slightly open by events in this year, that part of my personality needs to be given some kind of direction or it becomes very destructive. (And yes, I also need to stop telling myself I am a control freak.) So Swamiji's little sentence dropped neatly into my mind, provoking an "Oh yes. You're so right! How did I miss that one?" kind of reaction. Because when I think about it that way it is immensely comforting. We really are all in it together and there is no escape :-).

It makes not the slightest bit of difference whether we are rich, poor, enlightened or complete control freaks; we will all trip our way off this mortal coil at some point and we have very little control over when that will be (barring downright stupid behaviour of course). Something in me released at that point and I feel a lot better. Her follow-up line in case I needed clarification was equally delightful: "It is a one way street and we are all heading the same way. It's just that some of us are going at different speeds from others. Get used to that thought." I love these cheery reminders that we are mortal; it is good to be positive and have dreams and goals, but I think it is very easy to start living in and for the future – including the things we dread – instead of the now. Either that or dwell too heavily in the past. How much do we miss by becoming lost in our thoughts, allowing them to take over like rowdy schoolboys on a day out? That feeling of driving from 'A' to 'B' and getting there without any memory of the journey. Letting worries about the future spoil the gifts of the present. I decided that I don't want to live like that anymore and just the decision to live each moment is helping me feel better and a bit less 'lost' than I was. I have decided that before of course – readers of this blog will know this is nothing new – but I need to remind myself of it constantly or I get lost in concerns about the future and forget it all again. My apologies to those of you who don't need reminding and are very ably living in the moment.

In pursuance of this thought I am currently reading Full Catastrophe Living by Jon Kabat-Zinn, which is a guide to coping with stress and illness with mindfulness techniques. I love Thich Nhat Hanh to bits but sometimes I need a more Western approach to these things. Jon quotes Nadine Stair, an 85 year-old lady, at the beginning of the book:

Oh, I've had my moments, and if I had to do it all over again, I'd have more of them. In fact I'd try to have nothing else. Just moments, one after another, instead of living so many years ahead of each day.

Isn't that just lovely? Stephen tells me this was one of the great self-help books of the eighties, a fact which clearly passed me by. The title is somewhat off-putting, but the author explains it by quoting Zorba the Greek, when asked whether he had been married: "Am I not a man? Of course I have been married. Wife, house, kids....the full catastrophe!" It embraces beautifully the feeling that we have to live the whole thing, warts and all. It's just that some bits are more warty than others.

I haven't been able to have the PET scan yet due to a cold, which I think has finally gone. Many thanks to all the kind people who have been gently enquiring whether I've had the results back, but no, as I haven't been yet. After two rescheduled appointments I am due in tomorrow (Wednesday) at 8.30am. It is always tricky timing these things as I can't eat for six hours before, then the whole procedure takes about an hour and a half after that, as I have to go and sit in my little cubicle waiting patiently to become fully radioactive before the serious fun of the scanning starts. The first appointment was for noon, which meant I could get up very early to have breakfast if I wanted to. Hmm. That was a tough call, so I was quite glad when I had to cancel it. The second one was for 3.30 in the afternoon, so I could have filled my face right up until 9.30am. Not bad. I think I have got the best of the lot tomorrow though – an 8.30 appointment means I can leap straight out of bed and get involved before I have a chance to get really achingly hungry. Then I can go back home and enjoy a hearty breakfast.

I expect all this agonising about food seems a bit strange to most of you, but I have some catching up to do and planning meals, especially the timing, is really important in getting my strength back. My sense of taste has returned for most foods, as has my appetite, and I am eating full-sized meals now but I find it hard to go for long without topping up the tank – hence my anxiety about six hours without food! On the exercise front, despite really not feeling much like it most days I usually manage to exercise enough to get my heart rate up, which is the important part. I was greatly cheered by my progress on the Isle of Wight as it proved that the exercise does in fact make me feel better once I have got my breath back. Funny that. I am sure someone has been telling me that for years...

I am still finding it hard to take it all slowly, but I am finally starting to appreciate it is worth doing the job properly, albeit at the speed of a racing snail. I was reminded today of just how far I had come in this journey of survival and regeneration: I was at a dental appointment and heard about a lady who has recently been diagnosed with cancer. Just the mention of it brought everything flooding back to me as if it was yesterday, but even as I struggled to keep my composure I was able to offer some practical help and support; seeing the fear in someone's eyes reminded me of just how bad it all is at the beginning, and how every shred of empathy and support is welcome. Some people seem to almost shrug off their diagnosis and treatment, but it has run far deeper with me. In a recent interview Jennifer Saunders spoke briefly about her experience of breast cancer. Her attitude was very much that there is a lot of cancer about so deal with it and move on. No big issue there then. She was also told she was cured, which is a bit different. The power of the spoken word, huh? Jo Malone (of the lovely perfumes) also spoke of her experience but she put it differently, saying that she could have made it the book of her life but she has chosen for it only to be a chapter.

Nice. Having a Moon/Pluto conjunction in my chart definitely pushes me, unwillingly I feel, into darker waters than these two ladies, or maybe they aren't sharing their deeper feelings in public. Some time ago, and after a discussion on the darkest depths of Hades (I was in another cheerful mood!), my lovely friend Jennifer sent me a copy of Descent to the Goddess: A Way of Initiation for Women *by Sylvia Brinton Perera. I was struck by a passage which relates to sacrifice and energy exchange, and the way it brings about changes about which we don't have any choice; I realised how is summed up my feelings about my particular experience. She goes on to say:*

> *All we can know is that finding renewal and connection with the potent forces of the underworld will involve breaking up the old pattern... the death of a seemingly whole identity.*

And there you have it in a nutshell. As I meditate on releasing the old me and its patterns of illness, I welcome with an open heart the new, regenerated me, and an opportunity, theoretically, that is given to very few people to start over again. You see, always a silver lining.
I will be in touch just as soon as we get the PET scan results.
Margaret xx

Remission

It's a strange feeling, being on the other side of treatment. The whole period since December last year seems like a distant dream, whereas living through it felt like we had stumbled into someone else's nightmare. The funny thing is that I wasn't even expecting my consultant to have the results of the PET scan when we turned up for our scheduled appointment. I had the scan on the Wednesday and was told that it would take a week for the results to come through, so my sights were set pretty low, this being the NHS and everything. I was completely unprepared for the excited party atmosphere that prevailed in the office when I asked, very tentatively, if they were back yet. Funnily enough, neither Stephen or I mentioned them on the way to the hospital – he didn't want to bring it to my attention, and I had almost discounted them; as you will know from previous blogs I am very ambivalent about these things. The scan is only as good as the day it is taken, and things can change very rapidly. So, we had lots of hugs with both the lovely Joe and the lovely Lisa, and it wasn't until we got to the car that it hit me. As did the tears of course. Somehow it suddenly did matter very much that the computer said 'yes'. I didn't expect to feel such relief and happiness and I didn't quite know what to do with myself. There are still a lot of things to take into account though – I'm not off the hook yet. Despite arguing my case I think I will have to have the flu jab, as will Stephen and Matthew (my youngest son); they may well avoid having the flu themselves but they could be carriers and I could catch it that way. I know there are side effects and I also know that the vaccine is only effective for a particular strain each year, but the reality is that if I catch any kind of flu I could be very ill indeed – so I might have to give in.

My blood results were splendid, but I still can't go on a plane or mix with people en masse for many months to come as my immune system is very immature. To be honest, the amount of sneezes and coughs I've been hearing just in Sainsburys is enough to put me off. I usually wear a scarf as an accessory, and it comes in really useful when somebody is busy spreading their germs around; without wishing to put you off your food, every time somebody coughs or sneezes a great spray of bugs gets released which, if it happens to be close by, you are quite likely to walk through and inhale. Enter the scarf. I am able to hold it across my face and skulk through the potentially toxic cloud and hopefully exit the other side without having breathed anything in. Virgo moon people can be pretty fussy without any help like this. You can imagine mine is having a field day. The other obvious things are supermarket trolley handles and escalator rails. Isn't this jolly? I bet you won't want to leave the house until the flu season is over :-).

This also means we have had to cancel our Christmas party, which grieves me greatly. We have made the odd sortie to restaurants but I haven't managed to get together with a bunch of people for ages. Clearly it isn't going to happen for some while yet, either; we usually have about 40 to 50 people at our party, and the chance of someone bringing more than a bottle is extremely high at this time of the year. Oh well. Ho hum, as opposed to Ho!Ho!Ho! There will be other opportunities. To be honest, I am quite used to being a recluse now, although I am sure Stephen is champing at the bit. Now that my appetite is back with a vengeance we will be able to have people over in small disease-free groups and resuscitate our social skills that way. Sounds so inviting, doesn't it?

My appetite really is back, and I am so pleased and relieved. I am definitely not a 'foodie' but it is nice to enjoy my meals as there was a long period when everything smelt and tasted horrible. Well, most of this year, to be truthful. After many months of pushing teeny portions around my plate I am delighted to report that my taste buds are fully active and are capable even of appreciating Chardonnay again. That is a massive relief as the beautiful pink wineglass given to me by Cathy really does have to be filled with wine to get the full effect. I do still have reminders of those dark days. About once a week I suddenly become – as in feel and smell – really toxic and full of chemo. It seems to happen around the weekend, and I am trying to understand the pattern. I feel as though my pores are exuding chemo and I know it smells on my breath, which also affects my taste, although not as badly as when I was actually going through it. I have Liquid Zeolite drops, which are good for releasing toxins, and I take an Epsom salts bath (along with a few drops of essential oil) and that seems to help. I am curious to know what this is though and why it happens. I questioned Joe about it and he said it isn't toxicity. He said that all the toxins were out of my system 24 hours after the last chemo dose – they wouldn't be putting brand new stem cells into a toxic environment as that would be plain silly and very counter-productive. And clearly, according to the scan, the transplant has done its job. What he said is that as the organs replace themselves they are in effect casting off old cells, which I guess happens all the time with everybody, but in my case those cells have the remains of the chemicals in them. I don't know. The rest of the time I don't feel toxic, and my strength is coming back in leaps and bounds. Any enlightened souls out there, please – enlighten me.

I am really looking forward to getting properly fit again. I can't go to steam rooms or swimming pools until after the flu season, which is something else I hadn't thought about, so I need to just appreciate the things I can do. One of which is running, although I would hardly class myself as a proper runner, my get-out being that I am built for speed rather than distance. The furthest I ever managed was 5 miles (after a lot of practice) and I really thought I was going to die. Which is actually brilliant, because, in line with my cardinal personality, it means I don't have to spend a long time doing it to feel the benefit. I know people who don't even warm up until after 5k, so they then have to run an awful lot further than that to get any benefit. So I'm quite pleased actually. I can get out in the fresh air, have a nice little run of, say half an hour absolute max, preferably less, do a bit of stretching, then I'm ready to move on to something else, job done...

... And as an end note to the whole process I find that I did have some conflicting feelings after the meeting with Joe last week. We were all happily hugging and cheerfully bouncing round the room, but I had such a conflict in my heart. I remember vividly the period when I was considering chucking in the chemo to go to India for an ayurvedic detox. Joe and Swamiji talked me out of it, saying that the cancer was so aggressive that I could not risk a single cell being left behind – which ayurveda couldn't guarantee, but which modern medicine could – although the trade-off could be huge in terms of damaged organs and a possible relapse. Now, as I am through the other side of it, I am obviously delighted that we got the best possible result, but I feel strange having been helped, nay, saved, by something I hated so much, and against which I spoke so vociferously. I don't have an answer to this – it is another wonderful occasion where because this is a blog I can just say what I am thinking and be confused about my feelings and it is all perfectly acceptable. I am not deluded enough to think this is necessarily it – all over *bar the shouting. I have read a lot of stuff which suggests that the very act of having chemo locks you into the Big Pharma system; once you have had chemo the likelihood that you will need it again is very high, so they have a guaranteed customer base to milk. That makes me very cross, but at this point I am also strangely grateful because at least for this moment I am free of cancer. I suppose what it takes me back to is that we can't know the future. I might be absolutely fine for decades to come and die of old age. Wouldn't that be wonderful?*

Thank you so much for sharing my latest musings

Wishing you all good health

Mxx

Epilogue

It is all very strange. The blogs have definitely had their own lives in all this and when I got to the end of the book I found that the Epilogue also had its own sense of timing. I had already written about life after chemo and diet and lifestyle and all that stuff; the manuscript was finished and we were nearly ready to submit it, then my throat started feeling really uncomfortable. The story clearly wasn't finished.

We were due to go to an appointment with Joe and I thought I really should mention my throat, but part of me was thinking, 'Noooooo! I want this all to finish. If I ignore it, it will go away.' Which of course it never will. So I bowed to the pressure of some very sensible people – thank you Stephen and Judy – and confessed to Joe that I wasn't feeling great. It was all kind of upsetting as we were called in to the appointment to find he had a medical student sitting in for training. That wouldn't usually have bothered me, but Joe was really bouncy and excitable and stood up to greet us saying, "So this is brilliant, you are back at work full time! This is how it should be!"

I felt really horrible and like I was letting the side down when I confessed that my throat felt strange and that I really did want someone to shove a camera or something down it to make sure that I was still cancer free. Joe was brilliant, and without even changing pace arranged for my appointment with ENT to do their bit with their cameras whilst being very positive that my next appointment with him would now be in four months time. Wow! Sort of freedom after the throat is sorted out then.

My appointment with ENT arrived within a few days and I couldn't believe it. Same consultant, same hospital, almost the same day and time as my original one two years ago. There was the most awful and horrible sense of déjà vu.

Dr Emma King did in fact remember me and couldn't believe we last met as much as two years ago. After a quick look at my throat she said that my tonsils were abnormal and that I should either have them out or have a biopsy. I decided on the biopsy as I still see my tonsils as my early warning system, but inside I was so worried I felt sick. Please, not again.

Five days later, same hospital, same clinic, same surgeon. What was going to happen this time ?

I came round from the anaesthetic and the surgeon was there to tell me that he hadn't found anything unusual. I can't even begin to tell you how good that felt.

Two weeks later we went for the follow-up appointment with Emma King, and here was the best bit: she greeted us with a huge smile. "I have the best news," she said. "It is fine. All clear. I am so happy for you. Go home and have a lovely, lovely Christmas."

"Yes!" I said, deeply grateful. "We will. Thank you. And I can finally finish my book!" Her smile in response to that lit up the room even though she had no idea of her part in it.

So there it is. The beginning and the end. Two astoundingly good doctors, an amazingly compassionate team of medical staff, and a new, bionic body sandwiched in between.

To quote myself from the previous blog (which I appreciate is probably really bad form, but it is my book so I can), it would be tempting to feel a teeny bit like it is 'job done'. But of course it isn't. Life post-cancer (for me, at any rate), is a whole different undertaking from a pre-cancer, or a never-having-cancer-life in which one reads about, and is generally a bit bothered by the constant reminders to lose weight, drink less, exercise more, eat more veg, eat less sugar, eat fewer carbs etc. but never actually does much about it. It isn't until an illness actually hits that you think, 'Bugger, I really should have lost weight, drank less', blah, blah, blah, but it is all a bit late then. I was about to write that by then my body had already let me down, but that isn't quite right, is it? I let my body down because there were some areas I didn't pay attention to that could have done with some improvement. You can understand that I have done a good deal of agonising about how much I contributed to the cancer, and what other factors came into play that meant I would develop it when others in possibly the same situation didn't.

I think it is well known now that we all carry cancerous cells within us but not everybody goes on to develop the disease. If you think of the immune system being the advance guard that stops marauding cells from getting out of control, you definitely want the army to be as fit and strong as possible. I am sure I could have helped them a bit more, if I stop and think about it. A long time before I was aware of organic food and the dangers of pesticides, I used to eat tons of fruit, especially grapes, which I loved. I would drive into town in my lunch break and bring back lots of fruit, often from the market, thinking, 'food from market = straight from farm = GOOD food'. Sadly not the case at all as I now know it comes from the same wholesalers as supply the shops. Trouble was, a whole bag of grapes on the front seat was too much temptation as I drove back, and often most of them would be gone by the time I arrived at work. The fact they were unwashed did trouble me a bit at the time, but they were too delicious to resist. It is only now that I know that grapes, along with tomatoes, are the most contaminated crops of all, I can see how foolish that was. How much rubbish was I eating along with all the grapes and apples?

In a perverse way I could, even then, have been sowing the seeds of my illness whilst trying to be healthy, which I think is a dilemma we all face. At that stage of my life I was child-free, cycling to work most days and swimming twice a week. I thought I was doing a huge amount to stay healthy and who knows, maybe the grapes weren't to blame after all, or New Orleans, or playing as a child in a field that was over-cultivated and heavily fertilized after the war. Obviously I can never know. Although I wish I did, just for my own interest and peace of mind.

A very big lesson in all of this has been that I can't change my past or undo all the damage I might have done – as in countless episodes of the grape scenario – but I can certainly change the future. I have had crash courses in more therapies, diets, religious disciplines and methods of programming the mind for health/success/happiness (delete as appropriate) than I would have willingly explored in a whole lifetime, and for that I am very grateful. I can take a cornucopia of knowledge forward into the future and explore it at my leisure.

As I write this section it is 2 years since my original diagnosis, and the stem cell transplant and the events of 2013 seem like something that happened to another person; in a way I suppose, they did.

Apart from the fact that I am now a bionic woman, I feel as though I have moved on to a new level. The length of my illness gave me the opportunity to review what works and what doesn't at The Wessex Astrologer; looking back through the book where we record all the outgoing post I see that apart from the stem cell transplant incarceration there were only a few random weeks when I didn't put in an appearance for at least part of the time. It was slow going and sometimes probably the wrong thing to do, but I am so glad I had the business to keep me going. Just as I am so glad to have had Cathy to keep the business going! But my priorities have changed, and I want something different for myself now.

I love books and I love publishing, and hopefully I will continue to bring books into print for many years to come, but now I also love writing. I love the way that an idea starts from a tiny seed in my mind and grows into something with more form that I can communicate through the blog. The blog was absolutely a life-saver, but once it had served its purpose the challenge then became how to turn it into a book. That is now done, so after all these years of publishing books by other people I have finally written my own!

My thoughts go back several years to a conversation with the lovely Barnaby, who worked for me at the time. He asked why I was publishing everybody else and not writing my own book.

"Because I don't think I have anything to write about," I replied.

Me and my mouth!

Bibliography

Bays, Brandon. *The Journey*, Attria Books 2012.

Brinto Perera, Sylvia. *Descent to the Goddess*, Inner City Books 1981.

Castenada, Carlos. *The Wheel of Time*, Simon and Schuster 2001.

Dwoskin, Hale. *The Sedona Method Your Key to Lasting Happiness, Success, Peace and Emotional Well-being*, Element 2005.

Kabat-Zinn, Jon. *Full Catastrophe Living: How to cope with stress, pain and illness using mindfulness meditation* Piatkus 2013.

Neumann, Rachel. *Not Quite Nirvana*, Parallax Press 2013.

Nhat Hanh, Thich. *Fear: Essential Wisdom for Getting Through the Storm*, Rider 2012.

———— *The Art of Communicating*, Rider 2013.

———— *The Miracle of Mindfulness*, Rider 2008.

Moorjani, Anita. *Dying to Be Me*, Hay House 2012.

Ober, Clinton. *Earthing - The Most Important Health Discovery Ever?* Basic Health Publications 2010.

Sherwin, Jennie. *Intentional Healing: One Woman's Path to Higher Consciousness and Freedom from Environmental and Other Chronic Illnesses*. Changemakers Books 2012.

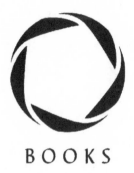

BOOKS

O is a symbol of the world, of oneness and unity; this eye represents knowledge and insight. We publish titles on general spirituality and living a spiritual life. We aim to inform and help you on your own journey in this life.

Visit our website: http://www.o-books.com

Find us on Facebook:
https://www.facebook.com/OBooks

Follow us on Twitter: @obooks